T0104850

THE SOSA MODEL FOR RADIOSURGERY

THE SOSA MODEL FOR RADIOSURGERY

A New Simple and More Accurate Method to Determine Radiosurgery Doses

FABIO VALENZUELA SOSA, MD

Copyright © 2015 by Fabio Valenzuela Sosa, MD.

Library of Congress Control Number:		2015914188
ISBN:	Softcover	978-1-5065-0768-2
	eBook	978-1-5065-0772-9

All rights reserved. No part of this book may be reproduced or transmitted in any form or by any means, electronic or mechanical, including photocopying, recording, or by any information storage and retrieval system, without permission in writing from the copyright owner.

The information, ideas, and suggestions in this book are not intended as a substitute for professional medical advice. Before following any suggestions contained in this book, you should consult your personal physician. Neither the author nor the publisher shall be liable or responsible for any loss or damage allegedly arising as a consequence of your use or application of any information or suggestions in this book.

Print information available on the last page.

Rev. date: 31/08/2015

To order additional copies of this book, contact:
Palibrio
1663 Liberty Drive
Suite 200
Bloomington, IN 47403
Toll Free from the U.S.A 877.407.5847
Toll Free from Mexico 01.800.288.2243
Toll Free from Spain 900.866.949
From other International locations +1.812.671.9757
Fax: 01.812.355.1576
orders@palibrio.com
711946

CONTENTS

AUTHOR'S BIOGRAPHICAL NOTE

Fabio Valenzuela Sosa was born in San Jose de los Llanos, small village of eastern Dominican Republic, in 1952. At an early age Fabio moved with his family to San Juan de la Maguana, located at the center of the first European settlement in the Americas and known as "the Dominican South's grain basket" because of its rich agriculture, where he lived until he graduated from high school.

Between 17 and 44, Fabio developed an intense and extensive academic career that gave him a Licensure in Physics at the Autonomous University of Santo Domingo, a Master in Physics at the University of Puerto Rico-Rio Piedras, a Fellowship in Medical Physics at the University of Wisconsin-Madison, a Master in Political Sciences at Pedro Henriquez Urena National University in Santo Domingo and a Doctorate in Medicine at the Santo Domingo Institute of Technology.

Fabio was a physics lecturer for 20 years at Pedro Henriquez Urena National University in Santo Domingo, where he was Director of the Physics Department between 1990 and 1996, and a lecturer at the Department of Political Sciences. He was pretty active in politics, being a member of the Dominican Liberation Party (DLP), founded by Juan Bosch, between 1978 and 1996. He was DLP vice Secretary of Professional Affairs between 1991 and 1996.

In 1996 Fabio relocated to the United States, where he has resided since, with his wife and two daughters. He completed a five year Radiation Oncology residency program at the University of Texas Health Science Center-San Antonio in 2001.

Since he completed his specialty, he has worked as a radiation oncologist in clinics and hospitals in the states of Iowa, New York, Texas and Wisconsin. He has worked during the last 10 years in several Gamma Knife centers. Fabio is Board Certified as radiation oncologist by the American Board of Radiology (ABR).

PROLOGUE

An authentic privilege was awarded to me when I was asked to present to you this theoretical effort of Fabio Valenzuela Sosa, MD, who happens to be a dear brother of mine.

It would be difficult for anybody to be objective when evaluating the intellectual production of a dear sibling, but in the case of the Sosa Model for Determination of Doses in Radiosurgery this difficulty is neutralized by the clarity of the objectives, the brilliancy of the ideas and the simplicity and elegance of the new methodology for figuring out doses presented to the radiosurgical community.

The Fabio Valenzuela Sosa that I have known since I was a child can be described as a renaissance man. He has scrutinized thoroughly the fields of basic, human and social sciences, while getting graduate diplomas in Physics, Medicine and Political Sciences with high academic honors. In the midst of an active career as radiation oncologist, Fabio keeps himself updated on the topics that he has studied during a lifetime to the level of fine details. While he approaches the age when retirement seems to be logic, Fabio's thirst of learning and hunger to teach all kinds of knowledge are, simply, insatiable.

Since 1996, when I first encountered a Gamma Knife unit, I have been fascinated by radiosurgery, to the point of forming part of the team that introduced the discipline to the Caribbean region. For longer than a decade I have found in Fabio a smart, candid advisor that has discussed with me the fundamental bases of his Sosa Model. It has been refreshing to me to see my older brother organizing his cleaver ideas in a book and presenting to the whole world reflections and observations that he has shared with me for longer than a decade.

I am glad to witness to you that, during my training and career in radiosurgery, the determination of doses was the most difficult and challenging task while developing my clinical skills in this fascinating specialty. After proofreading Fabio's Sosa Model, I can envision that the uncertainty and uneasiness that has been so far characteristic of the dose determination moment will disappear for the next generation of radiosurgeons if the Sosa Model or another one similar is adopted in the daily Gamma Knife practice. The Volume, Radioresistance and Eloquence scores would emerge as logic, reproducible, meaningful clinical parameters while studying a radiosurgical case and the adequate dose determination process would flow naturally. Clarity and objectivity would control what was during my training time immersed in the blurriness of doubt. I am confident that hundreds of radiosurgeons who could read Fabio's book will experience the same reassuring feeling.

We should pay respect to the rich data accumulated by 2 generations of radiosurgeons that have preceded us, but we have to respect also the right of our patients to have their radiosurgical doses determined in a logical, scientific, reproducible fashion, in tune with the amazing technical progress experienced by the Gamma Knife units since the first generation was unveiled in the 1960's. The Sosa Model is a positive step in reaching this goal.

This book is the result of a life dedicated to Physics and Radiation Oncology, produced with love and care for science, mixed with the fertile imagination of an authentic teacher capable of simplifying and making palatable to laymen arid scientific concepts.

I am convinced that the Sosa Model will become a useful tool for radiosurgical trainees, including neurosurgeons, neurooncologists, radiation oncologists, medical physicists and nurses; and even to patients and patients' relatives; because Fabio's language in this book is devoid of unnecessary technical lingua, making it accessible to the general public.

The author of this prologue expects that the brilliant ideas brought by Fabio to the radiosurgical table with the Sosa Model will have a positive impact in my specialty. I invite my colleagues of the whole world to read carefully the attractive prose in which the author wraps his revolutionary ideas and to let the power of these ideas enlighten and simplify Dr. Leksell's creation.

I assumed the delicate responsibility of supporting, from the neuroanatomical and neuroimaging standpoints, this laudable project endorsed by several decades of lecturing in neuroanatomy and neurosurgery at the Autonomous University of Santo Domingo and the Santo Domingo Institute of Technology medical schools, respectively. I hope that my contribution to this book matches the author's conceptual depth and professional excellence.

Santiago Valenzuela Sosa, MD; Neurosurgeon and Radiosurgeon; Clinica Corazones Unidos; Santo Domingo, Dominican Republic

May 2015

INTRODUCTION

Radiosurgery was, undoubtedly, one of the medical wonders invented during the XX century. The sole idea of treating a brain tumor without touching the cranium with a scalpel would have been considered like a science fiction proposition the second before a very bright brain in Sweden gave birth to what constitutes today the remedy for many intracranial abnormalities.

During the new millennium, radiosurgery has progressed to the point that one of the leading machine models that deliver radio surgical treatments has been named "Perfexion". This sole fact speaks volumes about the confidence of the radiosurgical industry in its capacity of enduring the test of time and continue, for generations to come, being the magic bullet that helps patients with intracranial tumors to cope with their disgrace.

In the midst of the big technologic accomplishments of radiosurgery, one worrisome fact projects its shade over this discipline: The theoretical base to determine the doses to be administered to brain tumors by machines that in all fairness deserve to be named "Perfexion" is, in the best scenario, shaky.

The main goal of this book is to present the Sosa Model, the product of the curious mind of a physicist converted by his circumstances to radiation oncologist, who has had the privilege of working for better than a decade in Gamma Knife Radiation Surgery (GKRS), considered by the majority of experts as today's gold standard for treatment of most patients in need of radiosurgery.

The first chapter of this compact book contains a brief summary of the history of Gamma Knife Radiation Surgery (GKRS) and Linac Based Radiation Surgery (LBRS), the two leading modalities in the specialty. The second chapter introduces the concept of Volume Score (VS), the third one the concept of Radioresistance Score (RS) and the fourth one the concept of Eloquence Score (ES). The fifth chapter builds Sosa Score (SS) based on the 3 previously presented scores, and the sixth one contains an MRI Mini Atlas of the brain that is used to apply the Sosa Model to better than a dozen clinical cases. This Mini Atlas is the exclusive creation of Santiago Valenzuela Sosa, MD, a gifted neurosurgeon, neuroanatomist and radiosurgeon with better than 3 decades of experience in Europe and the Americas. The final chapter is devoted to conclusions and reflections on the future of radiosurgery; in particular, to the urgent need of putting the accuracy of dose determination at the same level of the breathtaking accuracy in delivering those doses that has already been accomplished by the radiosurgery industry.

CHAPTER ONE

BRIEF HISTORICAL SUMMARY

Radiosurgery had its womb in the luminous brain of Swedish neurosurgeon Lars Leksell, who, confronted by tumors located in non-accessible loci inside the cranium, envisioned in the late 1940's a rudimentary set up of electrodes and probes that could be directed to the approximate location of the surgically unreachable intracranial tumors. Two decades of experimentation, with the assistance of physicists, allowed Dr. Leksell genius to give birth to the first Gamma Knife radio- surgical unit that started to treat patients in the Karolinska Institute of Stockholm, Sweden, in the late 1960's.

The Leksell invention, which in retrospect made him a deserving candidate to a Nobel Prize in Medicine who was never awarded, confronted the inertia that brilliant ideas usually find in the medical arena. It took 20 years to position the first dozen of GK units throughout the world. Argentina and England installed GK units before the University of Pittsburgh Medical Center inaugurated the first one in US soil in the late 1980's.

The introduction of a GK unit to the US market was a turning point in the history of the device. In a matter of a few years the new miracle of neurosurgery melted the ice of doubt that initially greeted it at the cathedral of modern medicine. A decade after its arrival to the US, GKRS units containing 201 Cobalt 60 sources, nested in a metallic helmet, all of them directed to the same point, were the gold standard of radiosurgery all over the world.

Approximately at the same time that Dr. Leksell invented GK, researchers in England built the first linear accelerator (Linac) unit prepared for treatment of cancers of different kinds, including brain cancers. Since the 1960's Linacs took over the US radiation oncology market, relegating the old external beam radiation Cobalt units to a corner of history.

The Linac units, eventually, became very sophisticated and accurate; at which point, during the late 1990's, the Linac industry decided to challenge the Gamma Knife industry as the optimal radiosurgical solution. A formidable goal to achieve, considering that GK units are capable of delivering intracranial doses with a spatial accuracy of less than a millimeter.

The field of radiosurgery has witnessed a fierce competition between GKRS and LBRS during the last 2 decades. GKRS continues to be the gold standard for most intracranial tumors not amenable to resection, but LBRS needs less physics logistics to function and is economically more viable than GKRS. In addition to this, LBRS, which is usually administered in several fractions, not in one fraction like GKRS is usually administered, has been considered so far safer in the treatment of tumors located in the vicinity of the optic apparatus and other delicate intracranial structures.

As of 2015, there are hundreds of GK units scattered over the world administering radiosurgery to tens of thousands of patients every year. It is difficult to figure out how many patients receive radiosurgery delivered by LBRS, but the number of Linac units able to perform this procedure is much higher than the number of GK units and the number of patients treated with this modality is thought to be considerably higher than those treated with GKRS.

CHAPTER TWO

VOLUME SCORE (VS)

During the spring of 2001 a radiation oncology senior resident, the author of this book, while doing a rotation in radiosurgery, had the privilege of participating, as an observer, in his first GKRS case.

A team formed by a neurosurgeon, a radiation oncologist, a medical physicist, a therapist and a nurse treated a middle aged male with 2 brain metastases from an adenocarcinoma of the lung primary.

Our senior resident was shocked to learn during his first exposure to GKRS that the tumor volume was to be evaluated in centimeters (cm), not in cubic centimeters (cc). One of the specialists explained to the resident that the doses to be used were going to be 20 Gy, prescribed to the 50% isodose line that would cover entirely the tumor of 1.20 cm maximum diameter; a "bigger" tumor of 2.10 cm maximum diameter would receive 16 Gy prescribed to the appropriate 50% isodose line. That meant that the maximum dose received by the tumor with 1.20 cm maximum diameter would be 40 Gy and the minimum dose would be 20 Gy. On the other hand, the "bigger" tumor of 2.10 cm maximum diameter would receive 32 Gy and 16 Gy, respectively, as maximum and minimum doses.

The specialist graciously explained that the "bigger" tumor had more neighboring structures like nerves, vessels and normal brain parenchyma, so it carried a bigger chance for toxicities as a result of the procedure; so, its dose should be lower than the one delivered to the "smaller" tumor. The patient was treated according to a protocol based on maximum diameter values and was sent to the recovery area in stable condition.

Our resident, still feeling the impact of having to understand and accept such a strange method of volume measurement using a linear unit like cm, stayed in the GK suite with the physicist after the procedure was completed and asked him if it was possible to obtain the volume in cubic centimeters (cc) of the 2 metastatic brain tumors that had been just radiated.

The physicist smiled with satisfaction and said "it will take this computer software 2 milliseconds to figure that out". The resident asked if he could copy the results, and the physicist consented as long as no personal information related to the patient was recorded.

The volume results were surprising to the physicist but not to the radiation oncology resident. The volume of the "bigger" tumor of 2.10cm maximum diameter was 0.52cc; and the volume of the "smaller" tumor of 1.20cm maximum diameter was 0.73cc. That day of the spring of 2001 our senior resident was convinced, as he is now, 14 years after he observed his first GKRS case, that the maximum diameter is a very unreliable measurement of a tumor volume.

Our resident asked the physicist if the discrepancy between maximum diameter and volume in the determination of tumor size was a frequent occurrence in Gamma Knife Radiation Surgery. The physicist shrugged his shoulders and with a dismissive tone counseled the resident: "If you are planning to work in the Gamma Knife business you will need to learn to think, when it comes to tumor volume, in terms of centimeters, never in terms of cubic centimeters. You have got to keep it simple, man…. There is no big theory in this field, just follow the cookbook".

The dismissive and patronizing tone used by the physicist counseling our resident operated as a challenge to a former medical physicist that decided to pursue a radiation oncologist career while doing a medical physics Fulbright fellowship under the direction of Dr. John Cameron, founder of the world's first medical physics department at the University of Wisconsin-Madison. This physicist, unknowingly, was the catalyst of the imaginative process that led to the concept of Volume Score for tumors treated with GKRS presented in this chapter.

To understand how the tumor with bigger maximum diameter could have had a smaller volume than the one with smaller maximum diameter is very easy. Just pick 2 of the many friends you have met in your life. One of them, rather low in stature but very obese, weighs 300 lb. The other one, of normal stature, higher than the obese friend and cachectic, weighs 100 lb. Which one would you say has a bigger volume? Of course the very obese, even if the maximum diameter of the cachectic friend, his height, is bigger.

The maximum diameter is a rather inaccurate surrogate for tumor volume and it is sad that as of 2015 many neurosurgeons and radiation oncologists involved in radiosurgery still use this inappropriate method to determine doses to be administered to a piece of brain or of other delicate intracranial structure of a human being.

It is very unfortunate that in an era where the volume of an intracranial tumor can be calculated in cubic centimeters (cc) in a few milliseconds by a computer connected to a GKRS software, radiation oncologists and neurosurgeons are caring about the maximum diameter and not about the volume of a tumor when deciding what dose will be administered during radiosurgery.

At the end of the day, could the inaccuracies associated with the evaluation of the volume of an intracranial tumor by means of its maximum diameter be relevant and have an impact in the treatment outcome? The answer to this question is a resounding YES.

If we administer 20 Gy to a tumor thinking, misguided by its maximum diameter, that it is SMALLER than a second tumor when its volume is in fact BIGGER, we are exposing the patient, unintentionally, to a higher risk of complications from a GKRS procedure. On the other hand, a tumor with overestimated size, as a result of the inaccurate maximum diameter method, could receive a dose LOWER than the one needed to attain local control.

Of note, the above discussed systemic errors in volume measurement most probably do not constitute medical malpractice, and will probably pass the test of a court of law. But they do NOT pass the test of conscience of an ethically suited physician. The maximum diameter model, simply, constitutes a WRONG model to figure out doses to be used in radiosurgery; a model that was justified during the 1960's, 1970's and 1980's; but is NOT justified in 2015.

In a few words, we need a new model reflective of the real tumor volume, not based on a misleading maximum diameter at the time of figuring out doses in radiosurgery. The Sosa Model is an attempt to correct this anomaly that can't be justified in any way today, when amazing technological advances have transformed the world in a global village.

In the Sosa Model, any tumor has a Volume Score (VS) dependent on what quartile it occupies in the range of possible volume values. The higher the quartile, the lower the Volume Score (VS) assigned.

What is the maximum value in cubic centimeters for an intracranial tumor treated with GKRS? The most accepted limit for the maximum diameter of a tumor treated with GKRS has been for a long time 3.00 cm. The tumor with higher volume with a maximum diameter of 3.00 cm would be one with spherical shape. No other shape will render a bigger volume than a sphere for a given maximum diameter. Refreshing our geometry, we will know that the volume of such a sphere is V= (Pi) x (D to the cube)/6 = (3.1416…) x (3x3x3)/6 = 14.14 cubic centimeters = 14.14 cc.

To make the quartile definition easier to remember, the Sosa Model approximates the volume of the biggest tumor considered by the majority of experts amenable to

GKRS to 14.00 cc. That will allow us to allocate the tumor volumes in 4 quartiles with the following Volume Scores:

Volume Score (VS)4 = Tumors 0.01 cc to 3.50 cc (1st Quartile).
Volume Score (VS)3 = Tumors 3.51 cc to 7.00 cc (2nd Quartile).
Volume Score (VS)2 = Tumors 7.01 cc to 10.50 cc (3rd Quartile).
Volume Score (VS)1 = Tumors 10.51 cc and bigger (4th Quartile).

As you can see in the table above, the bigger the tumor volume quartile, the number of normal cells surrounding the tumor is bigger, as are the chances for radiation toxicities; hence, the lower the Volume Score (VS) will be.

As we have said before, most of the functioning GK units in the world have software capable of obtaining the tumor volume in cc. No calculations needed. No time consumed in this task. Simply, draw the tumor volume and click a key board. In less than a second you will obtain a value for the tumor volume and following the table shown above you will be able to assign a value for VS!

Some GKRS teams treat tumors up to a maximum diameter of 4.00 cm. An spherical tumor of 4.00 cm diameter would have an approximate volume of 33.51cc. Even if we do NOT consider this practice as standard, it is not uncommon today to find intracranial tumors bigger than 14.00 cc treated with radiosurgery. These teams can use the Volume Score table shown above to assign VS value.

Summarizing this chapter, the tumor volume in any location of the body, including the intracranial space, should be measured in volume units, not in linear units. The substitution of linear units like cm for well-seasoned volume units like cubic centimeters (cc) introduces an unnecessary inaccuracy in GKRS doses delivered to the most noble of all human organs: THE BRAIN; and to critical structures with which the brain shares the intracranial volume.

Common sense is inviting radiosurgeons to create a model that uses volume units, not distance units, to measure intracranial tumor volumes. This new model, the

Sosa Model or another one that proves to be superior to it, is a necessary step in the right direction in the management of many thousands of patients in need of GKRS and other radiosurgical techniques.

CHAPTER THREE

RADIORESISTANCE SCORE (RS)

Since the emergence of Gamma Knife Radiation Surgery (GKRS) as a formidable tool for the management of intracranial tumors not amenable to resection and for subtotally resected tumors, this discipline has ignored the laws of radiobiology. The "justification" for this modus operandi, which so far has been accepted with very few significant dissensions, is that intracranial tumors, trapped in the brain-blood barrier web, do not exhibit the radiobiological behavior that characterizes tumors located in the rest of the human body.

Something "magic", which has never been explained, and apparently does not require any confirmation, allows intracranial tumors to behave differently, and, this being the case, "well, case closed and no further discussion is needed".

The simplistic negation of the radiobiological principles inside the intracranial volume has been "justified" by the "absence" of sublethal tissue damage repair after the administration of doses in the range used in GKRS. This hypothesis, which has never been proven anywhere in retrospective or prospective trials, has become a sacrosanct "radiosurgical law". The weight of this "law" is so heavy that, until recently, the administration of GKRS in fractionated fashion has been considered ill-advised; because what would make fractionated GKRS feasible would be, precisely, the sublethal tissue damage repair phenomenon, one of the pillars of radiobiology, "not applicable to radiosurgery" according to the status quo.

But a lot of water has run under the bridge of GKRS since the late 1960's; and here, there and yonder, from time to time, anecdotal reports have surged in regional radiosurgical meetings that have opened the appetite of researchers trying to expand the borders of GKRS and include radiosurgical fractionation as a viable option for tumors located in very close proximity to the optical apparatus. This practice changing trend is exemplified by a recent report of an important South Korean GKRS Center (see Jee TK et al in References) that has concluded, after a median follow up of 38 months with 38 patients, that "fractionated GKRS is a safe and effective alternative to either surgery or fractionated Linac Based Radiation Surgery for selected benign lesions that are adjacent to the optic apparatus".

Synchronized with the well-organized evidence mentioned above that shows that fractionated GKRS is doable and effective in humans, a recent biological optimization model (see Andisheh et al in References) concluded that sublethal damage repair can be explained in radiosurgery by mathematical models and that "differences in repair kinetics of normal tissue and tumors can be used to find clinically optimized protocols". All of the sudden, by a coincidence, computational research and clinical data are calling, at the same time, for a new paradigm that would put GKRS in the radiobiology dominion.

The growing body of well-seasoned retrospective reports that show that fractionated GKRS is not only doable but safe and effective in regions thought to be prohibited to this modality until recently (see Nguyen JH et al in References), should be a call to the attention of the radiosurgical community worldwide regarding the need of connecting the dots of the recent clinical findings and promoting a shift in the theoretical paradigm under which our specialty has operated so far.

Mounting evidence is suggesting that there IS sublethal tissue damage repair in GKRS and that the idea of a blood barrier "tumor hiding place" that permits intracranial tumors to violate the principles of radiobiology needs to be challenged for the good of radiosurgery.

A new model that sees intracranial tumors as objects characterized by histology is needed. The Sosa Model aspires to be an initial step into the inexorable process of conciliating radiosurgery and radiobiology.

The Sosa Model (SM) views all intracranial tumors as entities with multiple characteristics, the most relevant of which are Volume, Histology and Location. The Volume, as it was established in the previous chapter, is represented in the SM by the Volume Score (VS); the Histology is represented by the tumor Radioresistance Score (RS). We will dedicate the next few pages to develop the concept of RS.

For better than five decades, pathologists, radiation oncologists and radiobiologists worked together in classifying tumor radiosensitivity using different models, of which two preeminent ones were formulated by Deacon et al and by Rubin et al (see References). These two groups based their radiosensitivity scales predominately on tumor histology.

What other factor could be more influential on the radiosensitivity of an intracranial tumor than its histologic features? Definitely, no other one would be more influential. This is why the Sosa Model takes the tumor's histology as the dominant factor at the time of grading its RADIORESISTANCE.

Deacon et al (see References) classified the tumors radiosensitivities in five distinct groups, from very radiosensitives (like lymphoma and neuroblastoma) to poorly radiosensitives (like melanoma, sarcoma and glioblastoma). Based on this well-seasoned classical radiobiological background, we can introduce to you RADIORESISTANCE as the inverse of radiosensitivity. Of note, this concept should not be mixed up with the radioresistance induced in tumors by either radiation therapy or chemotherapy.

The RADIORESISTANCE proposed by the Sosa Model is the innate one, the one that is associated to the tumor histologic features. If two patients have intracranial tumors with the same volume and location and different histologic types, the more RADIORESISTANT tumor will need a bigger dose to be rendered inactive. The most radiosensitive intracranial tumor will be the least RADIORESISTANT; the least radiosensitive tumor will, logically, be the most RADIORESISTANT.

Following the principles exposed above, we have classified malignant and benign intracranial tumors, primaries and metastatic, all together, in four groups of increasing RADIORESISTANCE, and have assigned an integer parameter named Radioresistance Score (RS) to each group:

Low Radioresistance	RS=1
Moderate Radioresistance	RS=2
High Radioresistance	RS=3
Very High Radioresistance	RS=4

Examples of tumors with RS=1: Lymphoma, Neuroblastoma, Medulloblastoma, Seminoma and Small Cell Carcinoma.

Examples of tumors with RS=2: Squamous Cell Carcinoma and Poorly Differentiated Adenocarcinoma.

Examples of tumors with RS=3: Well or Moderately Differentiated Adenocarcinoma, Meningioma, Adenoma and Schwannoma.

Examples of tumors with RS=4: Melanoma, Sarcoma, and Glioblastoma.

We remind the reader that we have assigned RS based only on histology. This means that while performing dose calculations for brain metastases we ignore the organ affected by the primary tumor. That brings to the discussion table the following question: Why we do not consider the primary tumor location as a factor when assigning RS to brain metastases?

In our view, once the metastatic cells depart their cribs they severed the umbilical cords that linked them to their primaries, leaving histology as the dominant factor to consider in calculating doses to control the metastatic tumor; that is why the Sosa Model ignores tumor primary site at the time of calculating doses for intracranial metastasis of different primary locations.

As we have said above, the status quo model for calculating radiosurgical doses is blind to histology. This model will hopefully fade away during the next generation of radiosurgeons. Why do we say hopefully? Well, just think that, according to the status quo, tumor cells of different histologic types seeded to the brain from dozens of organs are expected to behave identically in the intracranial space.

Following the status quo model for calculation of intracranial tumor doses, a brain metastasis seeded from a gastric sarcoma would have the same radioresistance as others seeded from a mediastinal lymphoma, from a small lung cell lung carcinoma, from an anal squamous cell carcinoma or from a testicular seminoma. To accept this model as valid in an era like ours, where histology constitutes a determinant factor in the decision making process in all branches of oncology, is not reasonable. It is just logic and fair to expect that the near future will witness the resolution of this radiosurgical theoretical deficit.

The author is aware of multiple reports that through several decades have claimed that GKRS is "blind to histology"; and of reports from prestigious GK Centers (see Flickinger et al in References) claiming that melanomas and renal cell carcinoma respond to GK radiation, when they are seeded to the brain and form metastases, better than lymphomas and small cell carcinomas.

Hundreds of retrospective reports contradicting each other, most of them from very recognized GK centers (see Woo HJ et al in References), have built the Data Babel that supports the status quo for calculating GKRS doses at this time. This status quo has been challenged by the increasing evidence that GKRS can be effectively and safely fractionated. This fact would not be possible if Gamma Knife rays would not obey the principles of radiobiology inside the cranium, including the sublethal tissue damage repair principle. So, we have to move on and propose new models and solutions, instead of defending "radiosurgical truths" that are negated by reality and common sense.

Summarizing this chapter, the Sosa Model for Dose Determination in Radiosurgery proposes that all intracranial tumors are built with cells characterized by a RADIORESISTANCE dependent on their histology and those tumors can be classified according to their RADIORESISTANCE. An integer parameter grading this quality, the Radioresistance Score (RS), is proposed by the author as part of a new and necessary paradigm that tries to determine in a more meaningful way the doses delivered to many thousands of human craniums that experience each year the disgrace of being flagellated by cancer.

CHAPTER FOUR

ELOQUENCE SCORE (ES)

Intracranial trauma caused by firearms constitutes one of the deadliest pandemics of XXI century. Factors fueling this catastrophic situation include sociopolitical unrest, crisis in the nuclear family model and laws that allow an uncontrolled trade of arms that makes in some countries easier for depressed juveniles to buy machine guns than to buy cigarettes.

When we are informed by a cable TV news report that a firearm attack has taken place a few minutes ago in another continent or in a city close to where we live and dozens of people have been injured and that a substantial portion of them have died, many of those deaths are usually associated to injuries localized in the intracranial volume.

It is interesting to observe that the survival of victims of intracranial trauma caused by firearms is associated with the LOCATION of the trauma. There are intracranial injuries loci that give the victims a good chance of not only surviving the traumatic event, but of preserving a good portion of intellectual, sensorial and motor abilities. On the other hand, there are other intracranial loci that, if impacted by trauma caused by firearms, carry a high probability of death or severe limitations in the motor, sensorial and intellectual functions. So, an intracranial injury caused by firearms is an authentic disgrace no matter what intracranial target was impacted during the trauma, but the magnitude of this disgrace is heavily dependent on the injury's locus.

When the same amount of radiation dose is delivered to different intracranial loci during GKRS procedures, the potential damage associated with the energy per unit mass inside the radiation target, which is what we define as DOSE, will depend on the location of the target hit by GKRS. We can, in this regard, consider the GK radiation a collection of around 200 different "minibullets" that converge in a mass inside the cranium that needs to be "controlled" or "inactivated". Every "minibullet" is shot by a Cobalt 60 source nested in a metallic helmet. They all shoot Gamma Rays that deposit energy very accurately inside the cranium with breathtaking spatial accuracy, fact that minimizes the damage caused by the Gamma Knife radiation therapy to the tissues neighboring the intracranial tumor.

To represent the capability of the tumor LOCATION of promoting neurological damage as a result of a radiosurgical procedure, we introduce the concept of ELOQUENCE, represented in the Sosa Model for Determination of Doses in Radiosurgery by the Eloquence Score (ES).

The Eloquence Score varies from a minimum of ONE to a maximum of FOUR. Tumors located in areas of the brain that control important intellectual or sensorial functions like the Broca Area, in charge of language, have an Eloquence Score of 1. Areas of the brain located far from any delicate structures are assigned an Eloquence Score of 4. So, the MORE Eloquent an area is, the SMALLER will be its Eloquence Score (ES); the less Eloquent the area is, the BIGGER the ES will be. The more eloquent the locus is, the higher the probability of neurologic toxicity and the lower the recommended GKRS dose will be. Tumors of the same histology and volume will receive different GKRS doses if their loci have different Eloquence Scores.

Neurosurgeons, Neuroanatomists and Neurologists are the specialists best suited for assigning Eloquence Scores to different intracranial loci. The Sosa Model inventor is lucky enough to have a brother with better than 30 years of experience in neurosurgery and neuroanatomy, and who is a practicing radiosurgeon. He shared his Model with that class of sibling and asked him to group different intracranial loci in 4 categories: High Eloquence, Moderate Eloquence, Low Eloquence and Very Low Eloquence. Here is the Table of Eloquence built by Santiago Valenzuela Sosa, MD.

AFTER THE NAME OF EACH STRUCTURE, IN PARENTHESIS, WE GIVE YOU, IN ROMAN NUMBER(S) THE FIGURE(S) AT THE END OF THIS CHAPTER WHERE YOU CAN LOCATE AND GET FAMILIARIZED WITH MOST OF THOSE STRUCTURES IN MRI CUTS. WE HOPE THIS CLINICAL TOOL, WHICH ENCAPSULATES DECADES OF CLINICAL EXPERIENCE IN NEUROANATOMY, NEUROSURGERY AND RADIOSURGERY OF ITS BUILDER SANTIAGO VALENZUELA SOSA MD, WILL HELP YOU TO CONSIDERABLY SIMPLIFY AND STANDARDIZE YOUR WORK INSIDE THE RADIOSURGERY CLINIC WHEN FIGURING OUT THE EXACT LOCATION OF THE RADIATION TARGET AND ITS ELOQUENCE.

HIGH ELOQUENCE (ES=1):

Broca Area (I) (Left Inferior Frontal Gyrus/Dominant Hemisphere(XXIV,XXXIII)), Wernicke Area (I), Primary Motor Areas(I), Primary Somesthetic Areas(I), Primary Visual Areas(VIII,XXI,XXXI,XLIII), Occipital Poles(XIV, XVI,XVII), Auditory Areas(XXX), Superior Parietal Gyri, Supramarginal Gyri(I), Angular Gyri(I), Paracentral Lobes(XIII, XV), First Temporal Gyri(IV), Fifth Temporal Gyri (Parahippocampal Gyri)(IV,XXXVII,XL,XLVIII), Lentiform Nuclei (Globi Pallidis, Putamina)(XII,XXII,LI), Caudate Nuclei(XII,XXIV,LI), Thalami(VIII, XII), Third Ventricle(X,XXIII,XXVII,XLI,XLVI), Fornix(XXI,XXV), Internal Capsules(Anterior Limbs, Genua, Posterior Limbs, Retrolentiform Parts)(XIX,XLIX,LI), Insulae(X,XVIII,XXXIII,XLI), Hippocampi(III,XXXIII,XXXVII,XXXIX,XLIV),   Entorhinal Areas(XXXIX,XL,XLIV), Amygdalae(III), Mammillary Bodies(XXV,XXXII), Hypothalamus(IV,XLIII,XLIV), Pituitary Stalk(VII,XXXII,L), PituitaryGland(V II,XXXII,XLV,LI), Adenohypophysis(XXXI), Neurohypophysis(XXXI), Monro

Foramina(XIII), Pineal Gland(XVI,XXIII,XXV), Habenular Trigoni(XXIII), Posterior Commisure(XXV), Midbrain(II,IV,XVII,XXXVI,XXXVIII,XLV,XLVIII,L), Aqueduct(V,XXI,XXVIII,XXXVI,XLIII), Pons(II,XXXVIII,XLV), Medulla Oblongata(II,VI,XXXVIII), Optic Nerves(III,XXXIV,XLVIII), Optic Chiasm(XXV,XXXII,L,LI), Optic Tracts (IV,XLIV,XLVI), Oculomotor Nerves(XXXIV,XLV), Trochlear Nerves(XXXVI), Trigeminal Nerves(XI,XXIX), Abducens Nerves, Facial Nerves(XXVI,XXXVII), Vestibulocochlear Nerves(XXVI,XXXVII), Labyrinths(XXVI,XLII), Accesory Nerves, Hypoglossal Nerves(XXXVIII), Cerebellar Tonsils(II), Cerebellar Nodule(VIII), Lingula(VIII,XXXVI,XLVIII), Culmen(III,VIII,XXXVI,XLVIII), Fourth Ventricle(II,XI,XXIX,XLV).

MODERATE ELOQUENCE (ES=2):

Premotor Areas(XX), Right Inferior Frontal Gyrus(XXXIII) (Non Dominant Hemisphere), Superior Frontal Gyri(XV,XXIV), Associative Visual Areas(III,XX), Corpus Callosum(VII,XV), Cingulate Gyri(VIII,XV), Anterior Commisure(XXV), Olfactory Nerves(XLVII), Cerebellar Hemispheres(II,VI,XXIX), Pontocerebellar Angles(XXVI), Perimesencephalic Cistern(XXXIX,XL,L), Petrous Bones(XXX,XLII) (Except Labyrinths=ES1(XXVI,XLII)), Petrous Apexes (XXVI), Cavernous Sinuses(XXVIII,XXIX,LI).

LOW ELOQUENCE (ES=3):

Frontal Interhemispheric Cystern(XXVII).

VERY LOW ELOQUENCE (ES=4):

Gyri Recti(IV,XLVII), Septum Pellucidum(XXIV,XLVI), Lateral Ventricles(Frontal(IX,XXXV), Temporal(V,XXVIII), Occipital(XXIII,XXVII,XLI) Horns and Collateral Trigoni(IX,XVIII)), Frontal Poles(XIV,XVI,XVIII), Temporal Poles(IV, XIV,XVII,XXIX), Falx Cerebri(XXXV), Tentorium Cerebelli(XIII,XXXVII,XLIII), Choroid Plexuses(XXII).

It is very important to note that many of the structures listed above are SINGULARS and others are BILATERAL. Bilateral structures are much easier to identify in TRANSVERSE MRI CUTS.

Santiago assigned the ES to different loci paying attention to the neurologic damage that could be caused to the tissue irradiated by GKRS and to other factors like vicinity of tumor to places like the entrance and exit of the third ventricle, where edema produced by GKRS could lead to obstructions in the cerebral spinal fluid that causes an elevation in the intracranial pressure, condition that carries an increased risk for a handful of clinical complications.

In summary, the Eloquence Score (ES) is an integer parameter that reflects the potential of structural and functional damage carried by the LOCATION of the GKRS target. ES=1 is assigned to High Eloquence loci. ES=4 is assigned to Very Low Eloquence loci. It is just logical that a delicate, HIGHLY ELOQUENT location is given a LOWER dose than a location far from delicate structures if both locations bear tumors of the same histology and volume. Isn't it?

Now that we are familiarized with the Volume, Radioresistance and Eloquence Scores (VS,RS,ES), we are ready to discuss and understand THE SOSA SCORE in the next chapter.

Figure I (look for shapes only)
BROCA AND WERNICKE AREAS= ES1

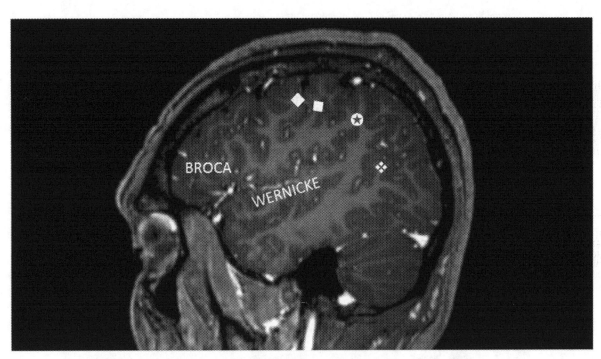

PRIMARY MOTOR AREA ◆, PRIMARY SOMESTHETIC AREA ■
SUPRAMARGINAL GYRUS ✪ ANGULAR GYRUS❖ = ES 1

Figure II
Fourth Ventricle✣, Midbrain ★, Pons❖ and Medulla Oblongata ◆
All the Above = ES1

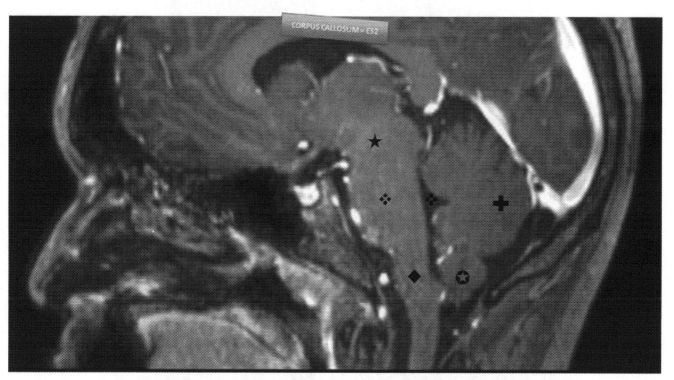

CEREBELLUM ✚ = ES2, CEREBELLAR TONSIL ✪ ES=1

★ Optic Nerve, ✪ Hippocampus, ⊙ Amygdala = ES1
Figure III

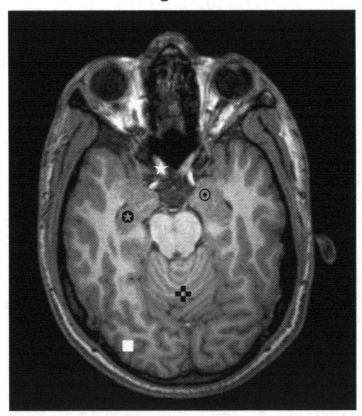

✛ Superior Cerebellar Vermis (Culmen)= ES1, ■Associative Visual Cortex= ES2

●Optic Tract, ◆Hypothalamus, ■5th Temporal Gyrus,
❖1st Temporal Gyrus, ✚Midbrain. = ES1

Figure IV

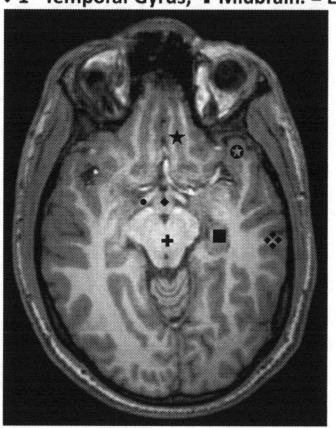

★Gyrus Rectus and ✪Temporal Pole = ES4

Figure V ⟹ AQUEDUCT = ES1

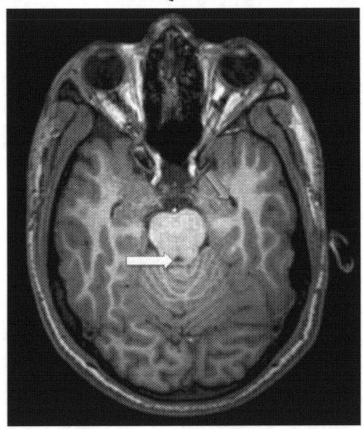

⟹ TEMPORAL HORN OF THE LATERAL VENTRICLE = ES4

❖MEDULLA OBLONGATA = ES1
Figure VI

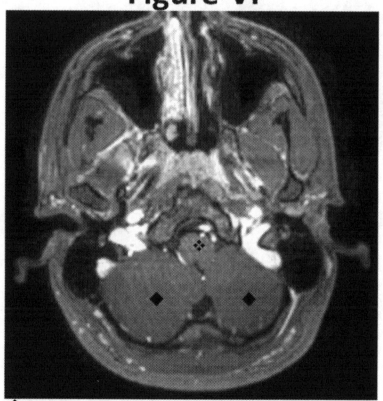

◆CEREBELLAR HEMISPHERES = ES2

⊙CORPUS CALLOSUM = ES2
Figure VII

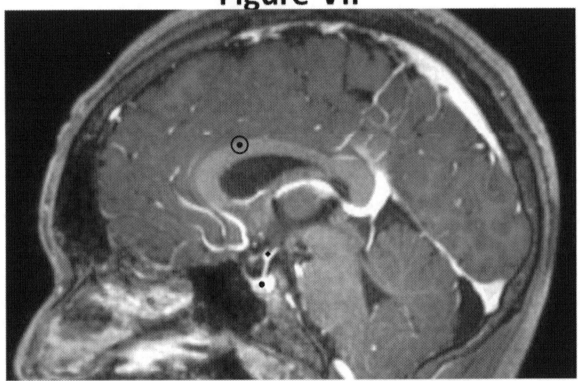

•PITUITARY GLAND, ◆PITUITARY STALK = ES1

✪ Thalamus and ◆ Primary Visual Area= ES1
Figure VIII   ✚ Cingulate Gyrus= ES2

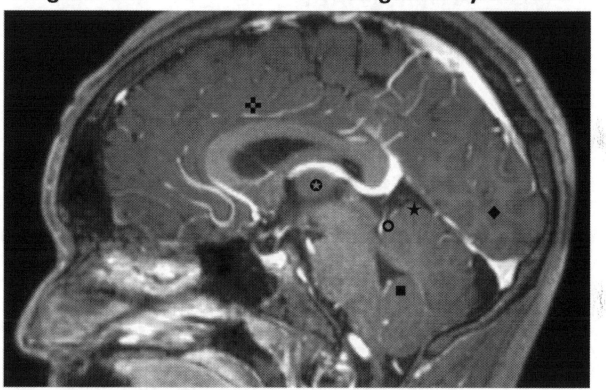

CEREBELLAR ■NODULE, ○LINGULA AND ★CULMEN= ES1

Figure IX

FRONTAL HORN= ES4

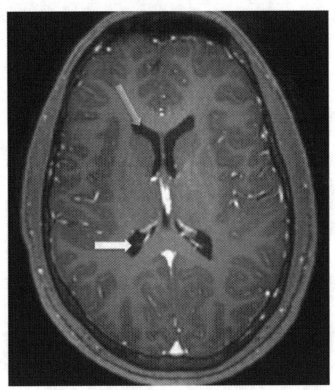

COLLATERAL TRIGONE= ES4

Figure X
◆INSULAE= ES1

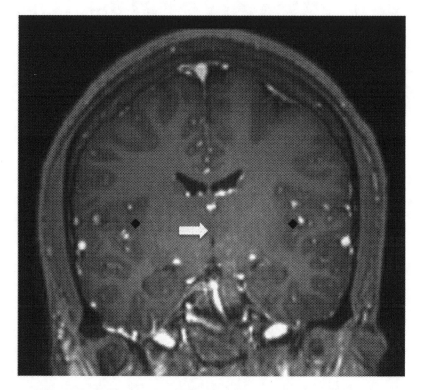

⇨ THIRD VENTRICLE= ES1

Figure XI
⇨ FOURTH VENTRICLE= ES1

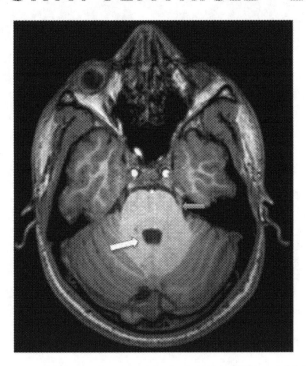

➡TRIGEMINAL NERVE= ES1

✪Caudate Nucleus, ■Thalamus=ES1
Figure XII

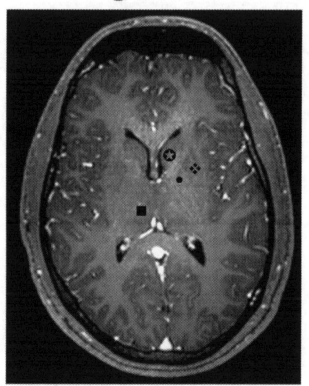

•Globus Pallidus, ❖Putamen= ES1

○Paracentral Lobe, ⇨Monro Foramen= ES1
Figure XIII

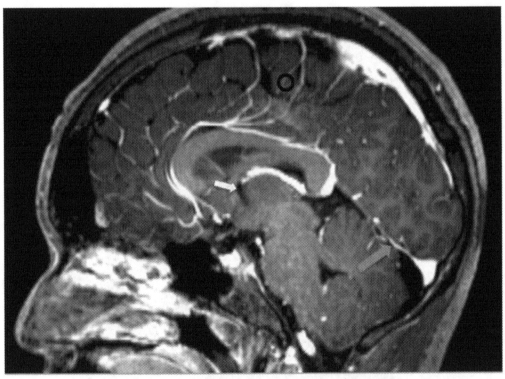

➡ Tentorium Cerebelli= ES4

Figure XIV
⟹ Occipital Pole= ES1

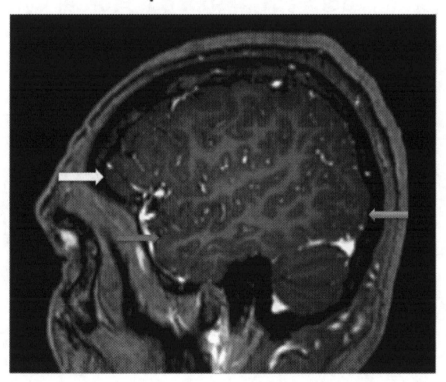

⟹ **Frontal Pole and** ⟹ **Temporal Pole= ES4**

Figure XV
✪ Paracentral Lobe= ES1, ■Superior Frontal Gyrus= ES2

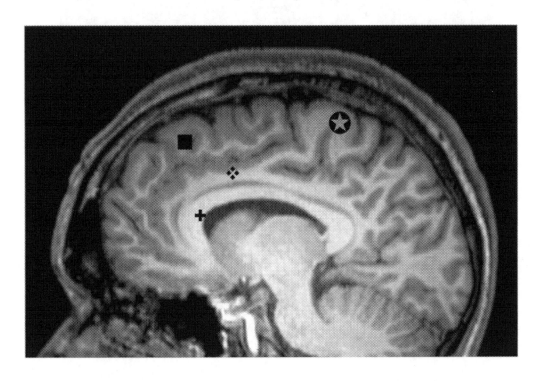

❖Cingulate Gyrus and ✚Corpus Callosum= ES2

OPineal Gland= ES1
Figure XVI

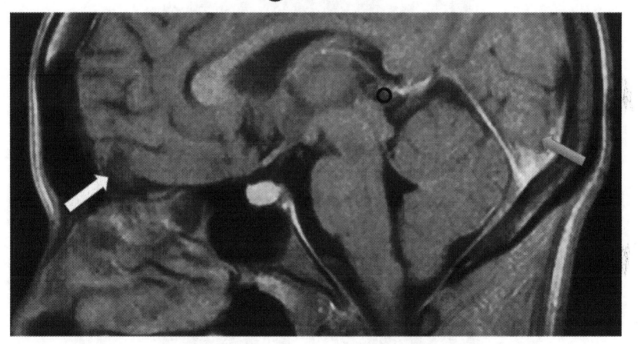

⇨ Frontal Pole= ES4, ⇨ Occipital Pole= ES1

Figure XVII

Occipital Pole= ES1

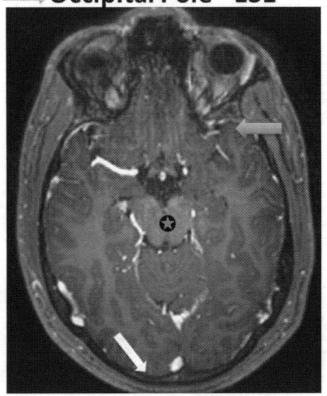

Temporal Pole= ES4, ✪ Midbrain= ES1

Figure XVIII
⟹ Collateral Trigone= ES4

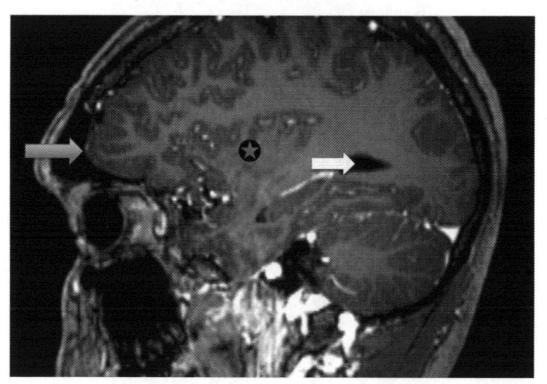

★ Insula= ES1,   ⟹ Frontal Pole= ES4

Figure XIX
Internal Capsule= ES1

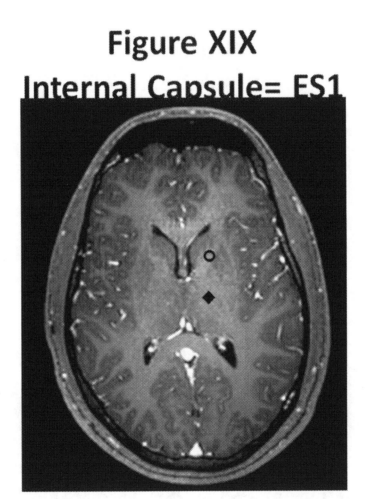

○Anterior Limb of Internal Capsule and ◆Posterior Limb of Internal Capsule= ES1

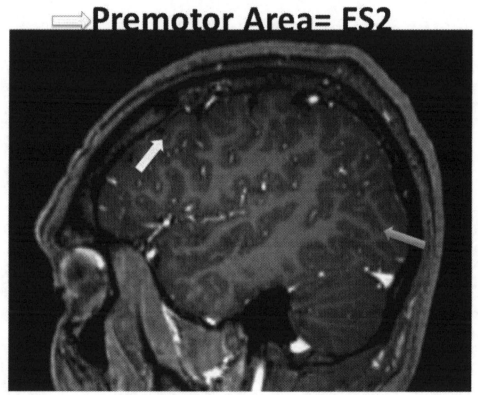

Figure XX
Premotor Area= ES2

Associative Visual Area= ES2

■Primary Visual Area= ES1
Figure XXI

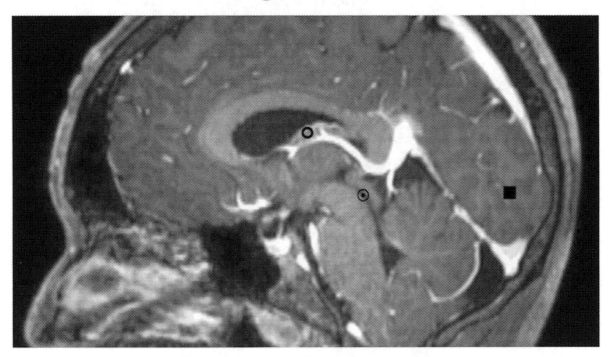

OFornix and ⊙Aqueduct= ES1

◆Globus Pallidus and ✪ Putamen= ES1
Figure XXII

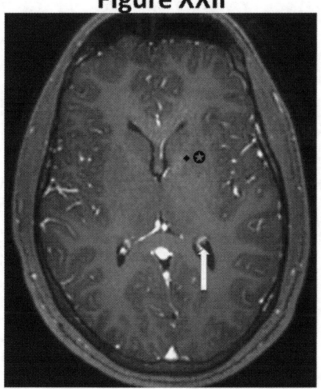

⇒ **Choroid Plexus= ES4**

• **Pineal Gland and** ➡ **Habenular Trigone= ES1**
Figure XXIII

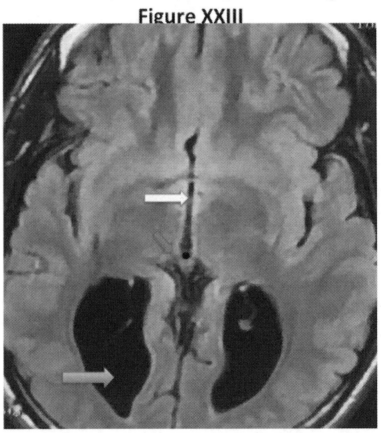

➡ Third Ventricle= ES1,   ➡ Occipital Horn of the Lateral Ventricle= ES4

⇨ Septum Pellucidum= ES4, ✪ Caudate Nucleus= ES1
Figure XXIV

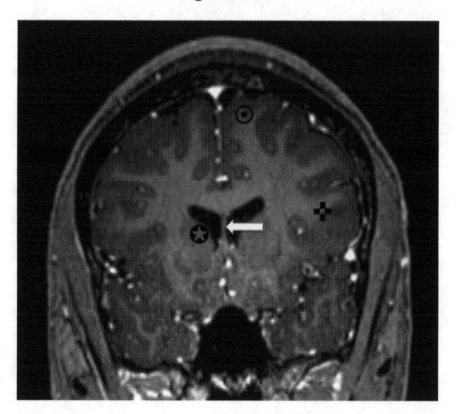

⊙ Left Superior Frontal Gyrus= ES2, ✚ Left Inferior Frontal Gyrus= ES1

⊙Fornix , •Optic Chiasm and ◆Mammillary Body= ES1
Figure XXV

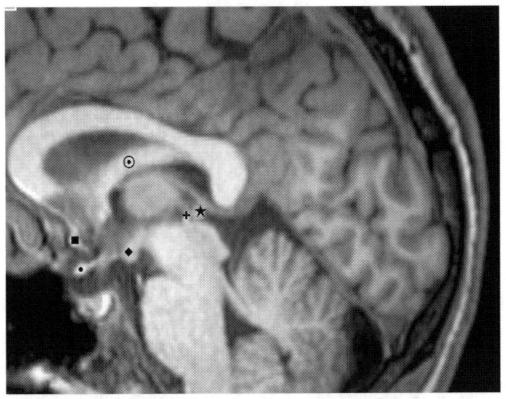

■Anterior Commissure= ES2, ✚Posterior Commissure and ★Pineal Gland= ES1

Pontocerebellar Angle= ES2, ✪ Facial and Vestibulocochlear Nerves= ES1
Figure XXVI

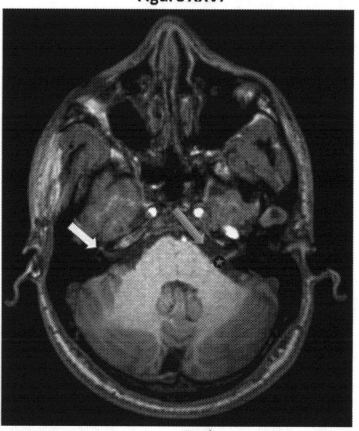

Labyrinth= ES1,   Petrous Apex= ES2

Frontal Interhemispheric Cistern= ES3, Figure XXVII   **Third Ventricle= ES1**

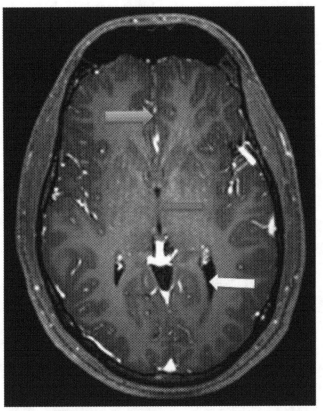

Occipital Horn of the Lateral Ventricle= ES4

Cavernous Sinus= ES2
Figure XXVIII

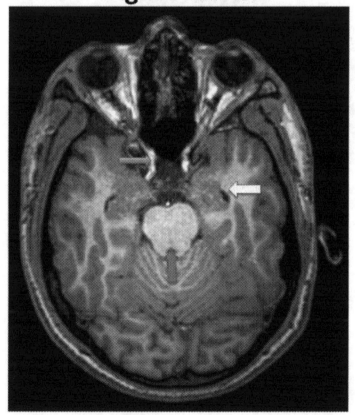

Temporal Horn of the Lateral Ventricle= ES4. Aqueduct= ES1

✪ Trigeminal Nerve= ES1, ⊙Cavernous Sinus= ES2
Figure XXIX

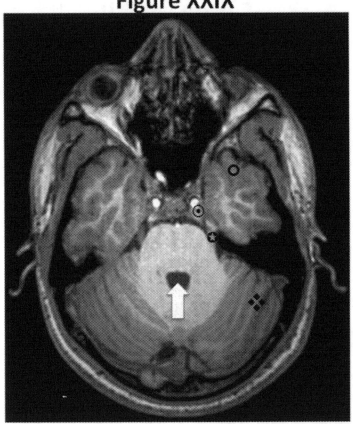

O Temporal Pole= ES4, ⇨Fourth Ventricle= ES1, ❖Cerebellar Hemisphere= ES2

O Auditory Area= ES1
Figure XXX

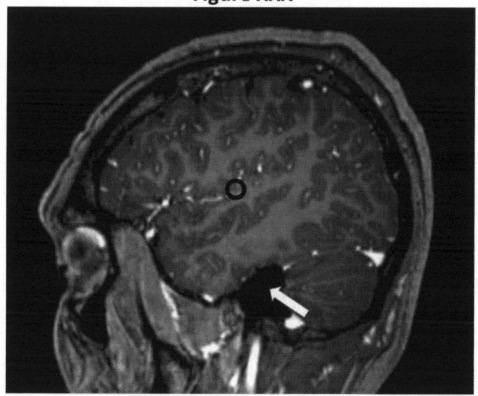

Petrous Bone= ES2

★ Adenohypophysis and ◆ Neurohypophysis= ES1
Figure XXXI

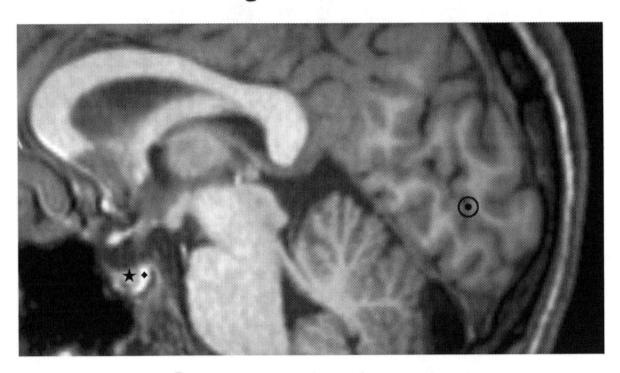

◉ Primary Visual Area= ES1

•Optic Chiasm and ◆Mammillary Body= ES1
Figure XXXII

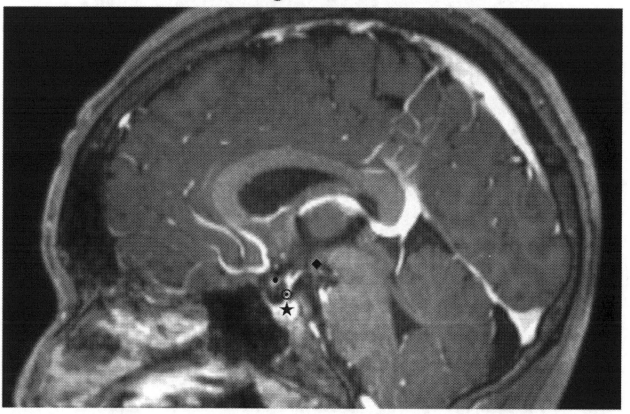

★Pituitary Gland and ⊙Pituitary Stalk= ES1

Right Inferior Frontal Gyrus= ES2, Insula= ES1
Figure XXXIII

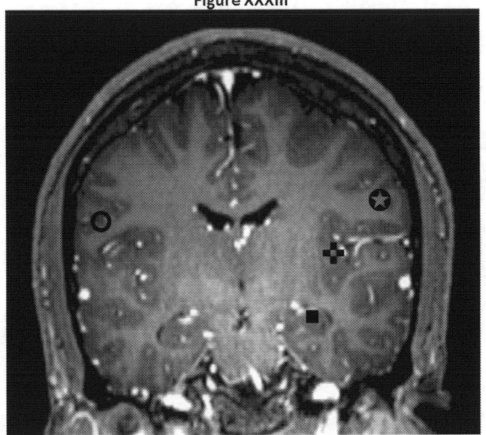

Left Inferior Frontal Gyrus= ES1, Hyppocampus= ES1

•Oculomotor Nerve= ES1
Figure XXXIV

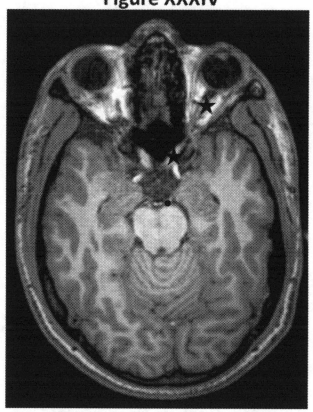

★ Optic Nerve= ES1

Falx Cerebri= ES4
Figure XXXV

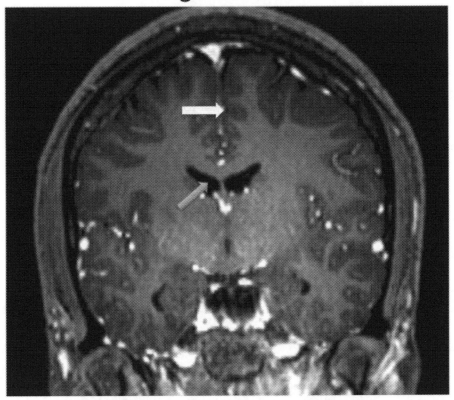

Frontal Horn of the Lateral Ventricle= ES4

✪ Midbrain and ⇨ Trochlear Nerve= ES1
Figure XXXVI

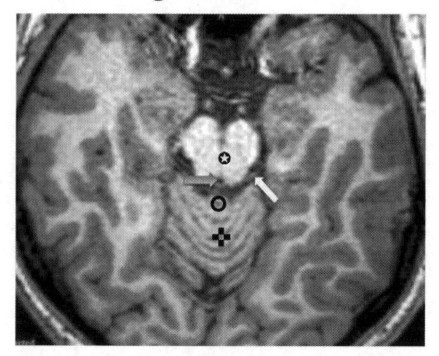

⇨ Aqueduct, ✚ Cerebellar Culmen and ⭕ Lingula= ES1

⭘Facial and Vestibulocochlear Nerves, ✚Parahippocampal Gyrus= ES1
Figure XXXVII

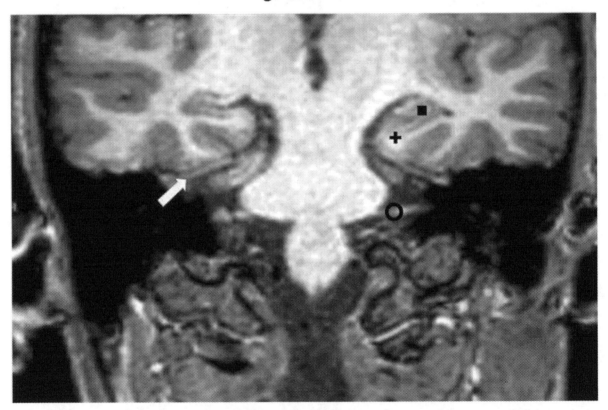

⮕Tentorium Cerebelli= ES4, ■Hippocampus= ES1

■ Midbrain and ⇨ Hypoglossal Nerve= ES1
Figure XXXVIII

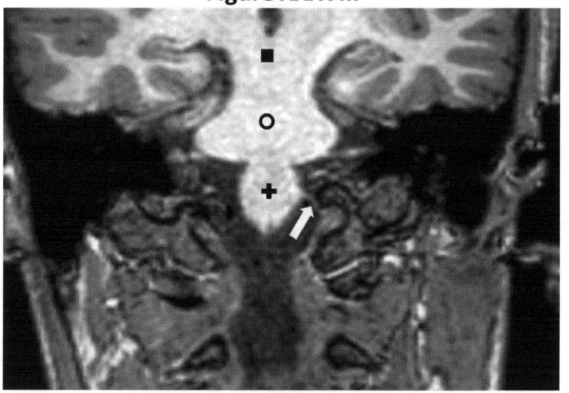

○ Pons and ✚ Medulla= ES1

✪Entorhinal Area and ◉Hippocampus= ES1
Figure XXXIX

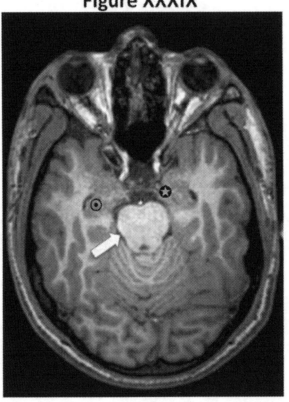

⇨ Perimesencephalic Cistern= ES2

✪ **Entorhinal Area and Parahippocampal Gyrus= ES1**
Figure XL

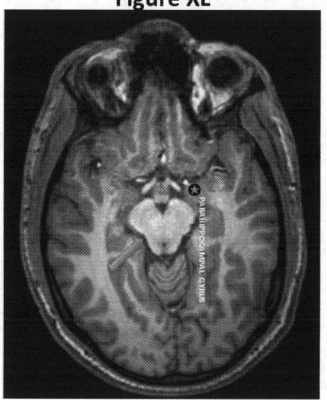

➡ **Perimesencephalic Cistern= ES2**

　　　　　　　FABIO VALENZUELA SOSA, MD

**Occipital Horn of the Lateral Ventricle= ES4
Figure XLI**

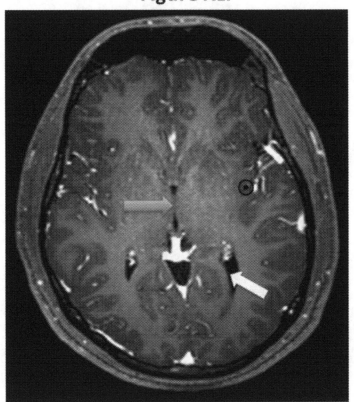

Third Ventricle and ⊙Insula= ES1

➡ Petrous Bone= ES2
Figure XLII

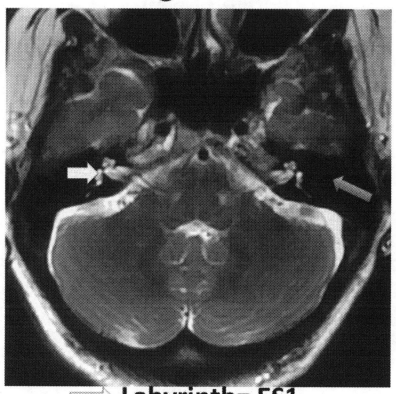

➡ Labyrinth= ES1

✪ Aqueduct= ES1, Tentorium Cerebelli= ES4
Figure XLIII

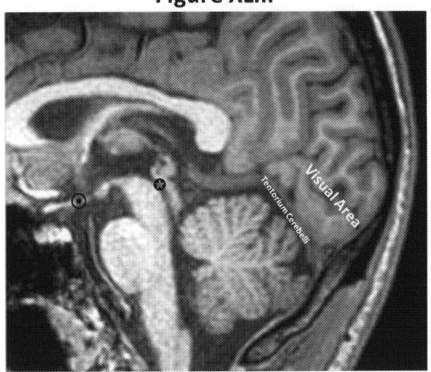

⊙ Hypothalamus and Visual Area= ES1

⊙Optic Tract= ES1
XLIV

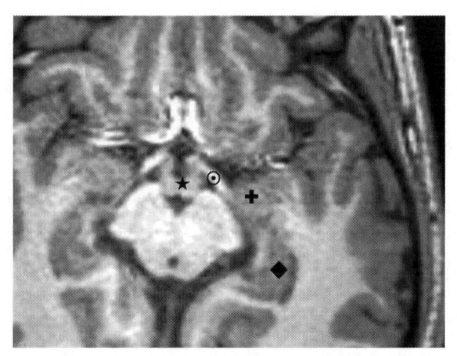

★Hypothalamus, ✚Entorhinal Area and ◆Hippocampus= ES1

✪ Pituitary Gland and ⊙ Oculomotor Nerve= ES1
Figure XLV

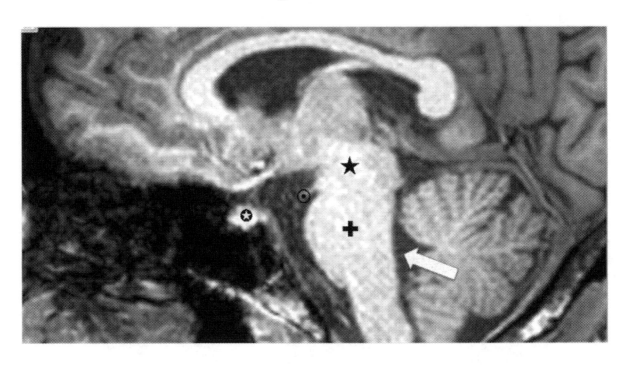

⇨ **Fourth Ventricle,** ✚ **Pons and** ★ **Midbrain= ES1**

•Optic Tract= ES1
Figure XLVI

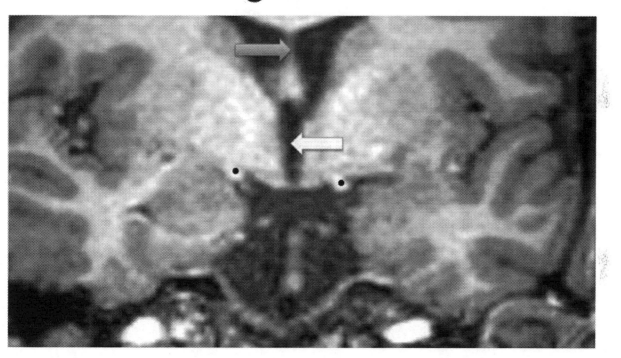

Third Ventricle= ES1, ⟹ Septum Pellucidum= ES4

Olfactory Nerve= ES2
XLVII

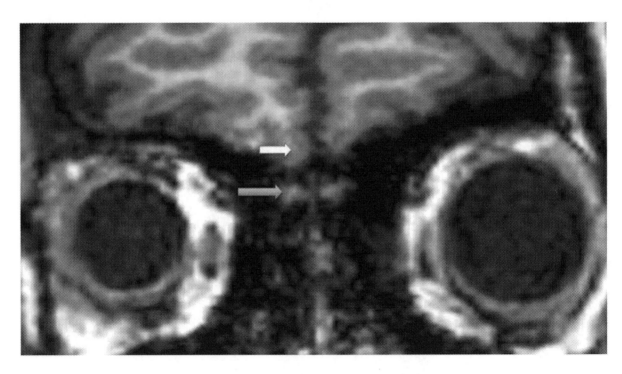

Gyrus Rectus= ES4

✪ Midbrain and ⊙ Optic Nerve= ES1
Figure XLVIII

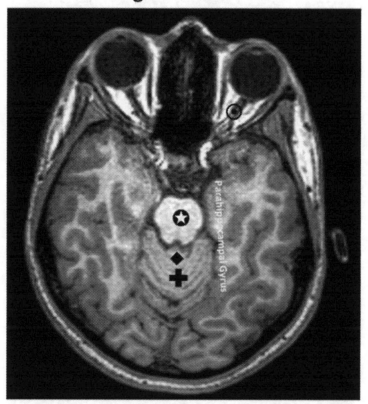

Parahippocampal Gyrus, ✚ Cerebellar Culmen and ◆ Lingula= ES1

Internal Capsule and Its 4 Portions= ES1
Figure XLIX

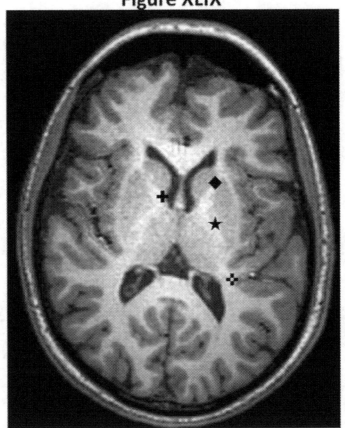

◆Anterior Limb,✚Genu, ★Posterior Limb, ✚Retrolentiform Part

✪ Optic Chiasm and ◆ Pituitary Stalk= ES1
Figure L

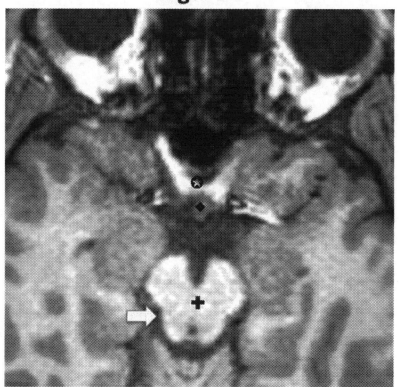

✚ Midbrain= ES1, ⇨ Perimesencephalic Cistern= ES2

⊙Pituitary Gland and ◆Optic Chiasm= ES1, ★Cavernous Sinus= ES2

Figure LI

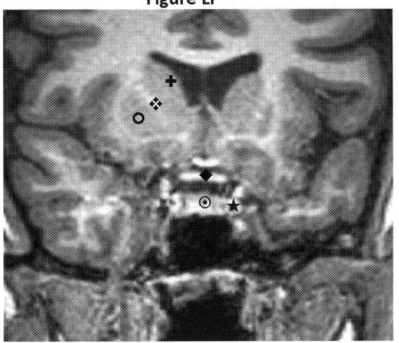

❖Internal Capsule, ⭕Lentiform Nucleus and ✚Caudate Nucleus= ES1

CHAPTER FIVE

SOSA SCORE (SS)

After presenting and discussing in detail the concepts of Volume Score (VS), Radioresistance Score (RS) and Eloquence Score (ES), we introduce Sosa Score (SS) as the sum of the three previously presented scores. In arithmetic language:

Sosa Score = Volume Score + Radioresistance Score + Eloquence Score

$$SS = VS + RS + ES$$

In the next few pages we will explain, with the help of two clinical examples, how useful SS can be in the determination of radiosurgical doses for tumors not located in close proximity to very delicate intracranial structures, like the optic and auditory apparatuses. These two clinical cases will also help us to build tables that can simplify a lot the challenging moment of assigning a Gamma Knife Radiation Surgery Dose to an intracranial tumor.

Example 1) A 70 year old gentleman with limited stage small cell carcinoma of the right lung treated a year ago with chemotherapy and radiation therapy and who has been in remission since completion of treatment, presents to his primary care practitioner complaining of difficulty in speech. An MRI of the brain is pertinent for a mass of 11.27 cc volume in the Broca area. The patient is referred to the Gamma Knife clinic for evaluation.

Solution:

Volume Score (VS) = 1 (Volume bigger than 10.50 cc).

Radioresistance Score (RS) = 1 (Small Cell Carcinomas are very radiosensitive).

Eloquence Score = 1 (The Broca area is very eloquent. It controls speech).

So...............Sosa Score (SS) = VS + RS + ES = 1 +1 + 1 = 3

WHAT DO WE DO WITH THIS NUMBER??

Let us think! What would be the minimum SS for a tumor?

Well............It would be, precisely, 3!!!!! Great.....By the way, do you know what is the minimum dose used in GKRS?

Well...... tumors that are not located in close proximity to the above mentioned very delicate structures, treated with doses lower than 13 Gy, are prone to local failure, according to multiple retrospective studies........

So.......The ideal dose for a tumor in the 4th Quartile of Volume (very big tumor), with very low Radioresistance and located in the very Eloquent Broca area would be 13 Gy!!!

We know that we are treating a tumor located in a very delicate area, with very low Radioresistance and with a big Volume. So we want to treat it with a dose as low as possible, BUT a dose that has a good chance of being EFFECTIVE; because, in terms of quality of life, tumor recurrence or tumor progression would be comparable with the worse complication. Are we on the same page??

Example 2) A 60 year old lady with multiple contraindications for craniotomy and history of high grade liposarcoma of the right arm was treated with surgery, radiation and chemotherapy 3 years ago. She presented a week ago to her primary care practitioner with worsening headaches that prompted an MRI that showed a 0.77 cc mass consistent with metastatic sarcoma located in an area of very low eloquence in the right cerebellar lobe. The patient is referred to your Gamma Knife Center for consideration of treatment. Please, figure out the GKRS recommended dose.

Solution:

SS= VS + RS + ES = 4 + 4 + 4 = 12

What is the maximum value for SS?? Of course it's 12!

And what would be the maximum safe dose recommended for small tumors of very resistant histology, located in an intracranial location of very low Eloquence??

Well.........When back when, a couple of decades ago, the maximum GKRS empirical dose was 24 Gy prescribed to 50% isodose, but that dose produced considerable toxicities in a minority of patients. Many radiosurgeons have moderated that top dose to 22 Gy trying to minimize toxicities. So we will recommend 22 Gy for this small, very resistant tumor located in an area of very low Eloquence.

Now, let us practice some interesting arithmetic!!

What is the difference between the maximum and the minimum doses prescribed in GKRS following the Sosa Model for tumors outside the optic and the auditory apparatuses neighborhoods?

Easy...........That would be 22 Gy – 13 Gy = 9Gy

And, what would be the difference between the maximum and the minimum values for the Sosa Score (SS)?

Easy...........12 – 3 = 9

Wow.......What a coincidence........... Man....You are tricking me.....

No tricks......This is a coincidence that makes the Sosa Score (SS) very easy to use in determining adequate doses for radiosurgery. Because for every single possible value of SS there is only ONE value of GKRS dose recommended; namely:

Sosa Score (SS)	GKRS Dose (prescribed to 50% isodose)
3	13
4	14
5	15
6	16
7	17
8	18
9	19
10	20
11	21
12	22

To make this "magic" process easier, the equation that connects Sosa Score (SS) and Dose to the vast majority of tumors, not located in close vicinity to critical structures as the optic and the auditory nerves, could not be simpler:

Dose (D) = Sosa Score (SS) + 10

$$D = SS + 10$$

It is worthwhile to note that even though there is only ONE Dose value for each SS value, there could be more than one combination of the triad (VS, RS, ES) resulting in a given value of SS. Let us build the list of all combinations compatible with the Sosa Model for GKRS Doses.

SS Value	Different combinations of (VS,RS,ES)
3	(1,1,1)
4	(2,1,1); (1,2,1); (1,1,2)
5	(2,2,1); (2,1,2); (1,2,2)
6	(2,2,2)

7	(3,2,2); (2,3,2); (2,2,3)
8	(3,3,2); (3,2,3); (2,3,3)
9	(3,3,3)
10	(4,3,3); (3,4,3); (3,3,4)
11	(4,4,3); (4,3,4); (3,4,4)
12	(4,4,4)

It is interesting to note that the SS values that are multiples of 3 (3,6,9,12) have only ONE possible combination of the triad (VS,RS,ES) and the SS values that are not multiple of 3 have THREE possible combinations.

The arithmetic symmetry that is present in all corners of the Sosa Score (SS) is a bonus to any specialist practicing radiosurgery. It makes his practice simple and enjoyable. No more guessing during determination of radiosurgery doses. Simply, obtain from your Gamma Knife console the tumor volume that will lead you to VS, determine RS using the tumor histology and determine ES using the tumor location; add those 3 values and you will obtain the Sosa Score (SS). To determine the GKRS recommended Dose simply add 10 to SS and you will have the Dose in Gy (of course prescribed to 50% isodose unless otherwise specified). As explained above, this equation does not apply to those tumors in close vicinity to critical structures like the auditory and optical apparatuses; in those cases the Sosa Model has to be tweaked a little bit not to violate the radiation tolerance of those structures. We will analyze a couple of those "out of the box situations" in the chapter dedicated to exemplify the application of the Sosa Model to different clinical settings.

What if you do not know the histologic grade of an adenocarcinoma because the biopsy sample was insufficient to determine it? In this case you follow the standard convention in all oncologic staging: Assume the lower stage or grade.

What if there is no biopsy in a case where it is indicated and the patient wants to have GKRS? In such a situation, make sure that you document the impossibility of obtaining the biopsy either because of technical difficulties, patient comorbidities, patient refusal or another reason, and determine the GKRS dose using your best clinical judgment as you did during the pre-Sosa Score era.

It is worthwhile at this point to note the usefulness of scores in different areas of medicine. To the memory come the Gleason Score used in management of prostate carcinoma and the Glasgow Score used to evaluate comatose patients. Why can't we, radiosurgery specialists, have a score, the Sosa Score (SS), to make our life easier at the time of determining radiosurgery doses while we base our clinical decisions in reliable, universally reproducible data, not in our mood at the time of delivering care to our patients? Why can't we have a Model that leaves everything unchanged in our practice, except for the blurriness and indecisiveness of the status quo at the time of determining doses that could be crucial for our patients' clinical outcomes?

It is worthwhile to invite the reader to note that the Sosa Model is not proposing to change the range of values of doses used in GKRS. It is simply proposing to connect those values to relevant clinical variables.

Summarizing this chapter, the Sosa Score is an elegant, very easy way of determining GKRS doses, based on objective data pertaining to intracranial tumors, that does not add any physical or financial burdens to either physicians or patients. For patients who are for any reason not able to be treated in a GK center and pursue Linac based radiosurgery, the standard conversions from GKRS to fractionated LBRS are expected to be used.

CHAPTER SIX

CLINICAL CASES DISCUSSION

After we have introduced to you in detail the Sosa Model, let's apply it to a group of real clinical cases. Unless otherwise specified, all doses are prescribed to the 50% isodose covering the tumor surface, and all patients are right handed.

----CASE 1----

History: A 59 year old lady presents to her family practitioner complaining of heaviness, tinnitus and hearing loss in the right ear, in addition to vertigo. The patient is referred to a neurology clinic, where an MRI of the brain is pertinent for a 1.90cc dominant mass (see Figures 1) consistent with right vestibular schwannoma. The patient is evaluated at the neurosurgery clinic, where, after discussing different therapeutic options, she declines to consider any craniotomy and consents to Gamma Knife Radiation Surgery (GKRS).

Dose Determination Using the Sosa Model: The most solid retrospective evidence presented so far (see Boari, et al in References) suggests that the maximum dose tolerated by the tumor location without increasing considerably auditory toxicity is 15 Gy. All vestibular schwannomas share the same Eloquence Score ES=1 and Radioresistance Score RS=3. In this particular case, Volume Score VS=4 (Tumor Volume smaller than 3.50cc) and Sosa Score is SS=VS+RS+ES=4+3+1= 8. The Recommended Dose by the Sosa Model will be D=15 Gy. Observe that 8 is the MAXIMUM value for Sosa Score in vestibular schwannomas.

Note that 15Gy is the MAXIMUM DOSE proven to be safe by the most reliable retrospective evidence available. If the tumor volume would have been 6.09 cc (between 3.51cc and 7.00 cc), the Sosa Score would have been SS=VS+RS+ES=3+3+1=7, and the Recommended Dose would have been 14 Gy.

If the tumor volume would have been 8.12 cc (between 7.01cc and 10.50 cc), the Sosa Score would have been SS=VS+RS+ES= 2+3+1=6 and the Recommended Dose would have been 13 Gy; and if the Tumor Volume would have been 12.12 cc (bigger than 10.50cc), the Sosa Score would have been SS=VS+RS+ES=1+3+1=5 and the Recommended Dose would have been 12 Gy.

Please, note that the Equation (D=SS+10) does not apply to this case. The maximum dose considered safe for vestibular schwannoma, based in retrospective experience, is not 22 Gy, maximum GKRS dose recommended for the majority of intracranial tumors located outside the optical and auditory apparatuses (see Sosa Score chapter), but 15 Gy. We summarize the Recommended Doses for Vestibular Schwannoma in this table:

Volume Score (VS)	Sosa Score (SS)	Recommended Dose (D)
1	5	12Gy
2	6	13Gy
3	7	14Gy
4	8	15Gy

59 y/o Lady, Right Side Hearing Loss, Tinnitus, Vertigo, "Dull feeling at the bottom of the ear".

Figure 1 a(Coronal Cut)   **VOLUME: 1.9CC (VS=4), RS= 3, ES= 1. SS= 8**

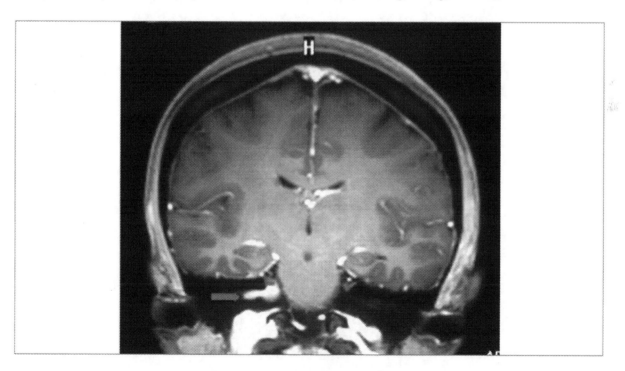

VESTIBULAR SCHWANNOMA

Figure 1b(Transverse Cut)

VESTIBULAR SCHWANNOMA

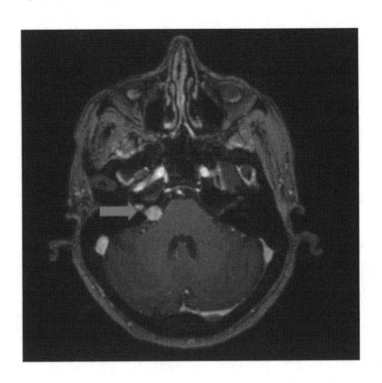

Figure 1c(Sagittal Cut)

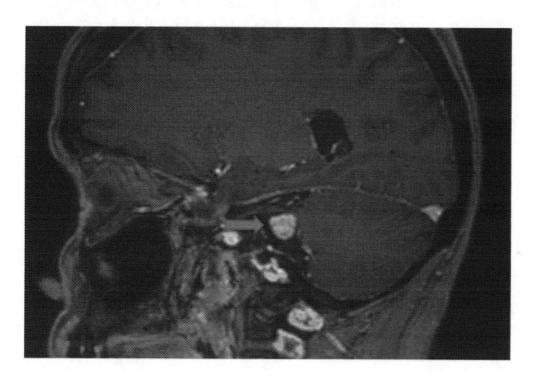

VESTIBULAR SCHWANNOMA

----CASE 2----

History: A 48 year old lady presents with sudden onset of seizures. The patient is taken to an emergency room, where an MRI of the brain (see Figures 2) is pertinent for a 1.43cc mass consistent with astrocytoma grade II located in the left supramarginal gyrus. The patient does not respond to multiple antiepileptic medications. She is not a craniotomy candidate secondary to multiple comorbidities and is referred to neurosurgery for consideration of GKRS.

Dose Determination Using the Sosa Model: The tumor volume of 1.43cc carries a Volume Score $VS=4$. Astrocytoma histology carries a Radioresistance Score $RS=3$. The left supramarginal gyrus carries an Eloquence Score $ES=1$. Sosa Score will be $SS=VS+RS+ES=4+3+1=8$. Recommended Dose will be $D=SS+10=8+10=18Gy$.

**Figure 2a(Sagittal Cut) 48 y/o Lady, Seizures
VOLUME=1.43cc (VS=4), ES= 1, RS= 3. SS= 8**

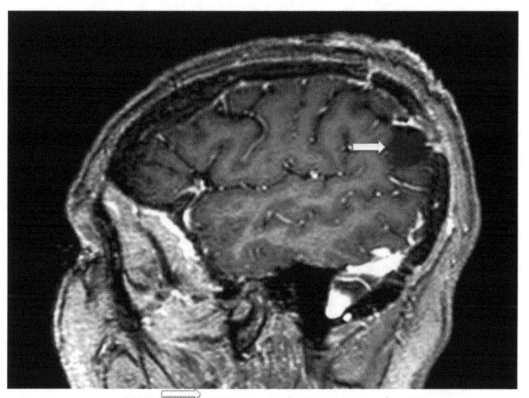

ASTROCYTOMA II – Left Supramarginal Gyrus

Figure 2b(Coronal Cut) ASTROCYTOMA II

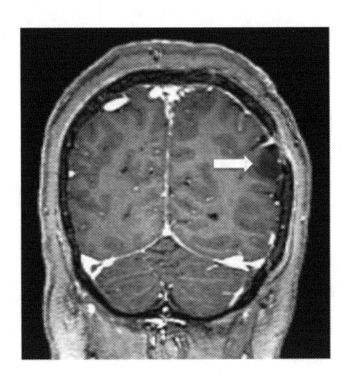

Figure 2c(Transverse Cut) ASTROCYTOMA II

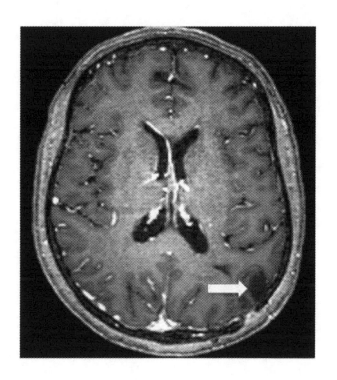

----CASE 3----

HISTORY: A 53 year old lady who was diagnosed and treated approximately 10 years ago for Stage IIIA left breast poorly differentiated adenocarcinoma re-presents to her primary MD complaining of left hemiparesis and headaches not controlled with over the counter pain killers. An MRI of the brain (see Figures 3) was pertinent for a 31.14 cc metastatic mass located in the right inferior frontal gyrus. The patient is referred to neurosurgery for evaluation for Gamma Knife Radiation Surgery (GKRS).

Dose Determination Using the Sosa Model: The patient's brain metastasis is bigger than 10.50 cc, so, the Volume Score VS=1. The Radioresistance Score of poorly differentiated adenocarcinoma is RS=2. The Eloquence Score of the right inferior frontal gyrus is ES=2. Sosa Score=VS+RS+ES=1+2+2=5. Recommended Dose will be D= SS+10=15Gy. Please, observe that ES=2 for the right inferior frontal gyrus, whereas the left inferior frontal gyrus has ES=1. Keep in mind that the Broca Area is located in the latter, not in the former. This is a case that illustrates perfectly the concept of DOMINANCE in the brain.

Figure 3a(Transverse Cut)

53 y/o Lady, Breast Cancer Evolving Since 10 years, Headache, Left Hemiparesis. Vol.: 31.14cc; VS=1, RS=2, ES=2. SS= 5

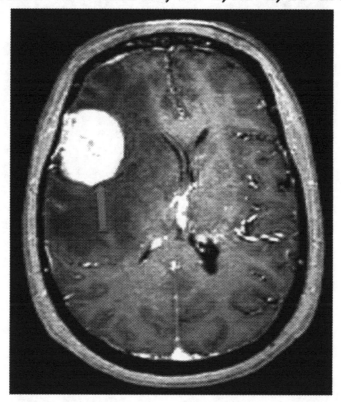

➡️ **BREAST CANCER METASTASIS – Right Inferior Frontal Gyrus**

Figure 3b(Coronal Cut)

BREAST CANCER METASTASIS

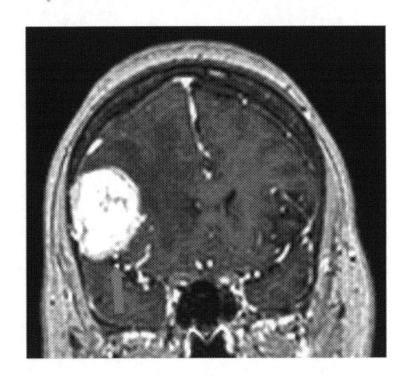

Figure 3c(Sagittal Cut)

BREAST CANCER METASTASIS

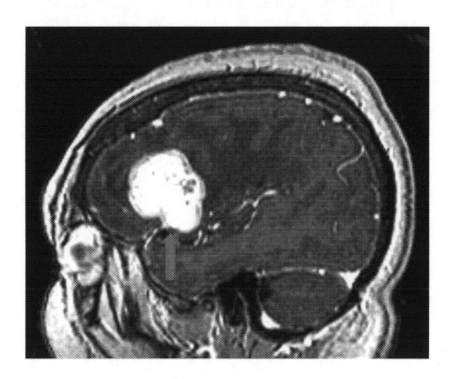

----CASE 4----

History: A 53 year old lady was diagnosed 4 months ago with a Stage IA right breast poorly differentiated adenocarcinoma that was treated with lumpectomy and sentinel lymph node biopsy. The tumor was ER negative, PR negative, Her2neu negative. The patient presents to receive the 2nd of 4 cycles anticipated of chemotherapy and relates to her medical oncologist that she has been having "balance problems" for the last 2 to 3 weeks. The medical oncologist requests an MRI of the brain (see Figures 4) that is pertinent for a dominant 4.84cc mass located in the left lower cerebellar hemisphere, very suspicious for metastasis from breast primary. The patient is referred to the neurosurgery clinic for consideration of GKRS.

Dose Determination Using the Sosa Model: The brain metastasis volume is 4.84cc (between 3.51cc and 7.00cc), so, the Volume Score VS=3. The histology is poorly differentiated adenocarcinoma, so the Radioresistance Score RS=2. The left lower cerebellar hemisphere's Eloquence Score is ES=2. Sosa Score will be SS=VS+RS+ES=3+2+2=7. The Recommended Dose will be= D=SS+10=7+10=17Gy.

Figure 4a(Transverse Cut)

53 y/o Lady. Breast Cancer on Chemotherapy. Ataxia.
Volume: 4.84cc.   VS=3, RS=2, ES=2. SS= 7

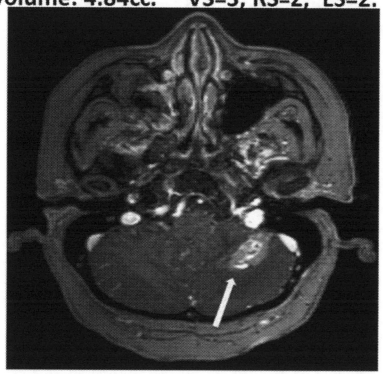

METASTASIS OF BREAST CANCER – Left Lower Cerebellar Hemisphere

Figure 4b(Coronal Cut)

METASTASIS OF BREAST CANCER

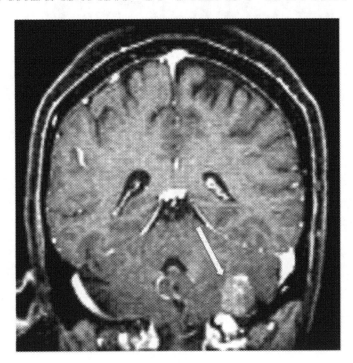

Figure 4c(Sagittal Cut)

METASTASIS OF BREAST CANCER

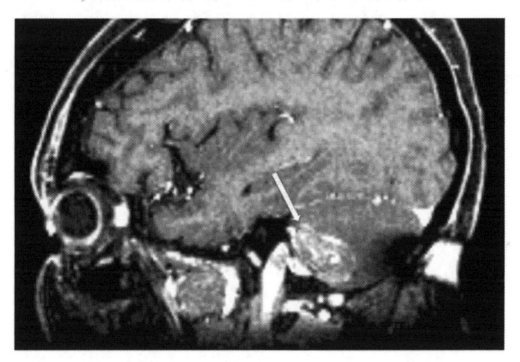

----CASE 5----

History: A 73 year old gentleman with 50 year smoking history of 2 packs of cigarettes a day was diagnosed 2 years ago with limited stage small cell lung carcinoma. The patient was treated with chemotherapy and radiotherapy with excellent response. He re-presented a week ago to his medical oncologist with left gaze diplopia. An MRI of the brain (see Figures 5) was pertinent for a dominant 8.28cc mass located in the left petrous apex consistent with metastatic small cell carcinoma to brain. The patient is referred to neurosurgery where he consents to GKRS.

Determination of Dose Using the Sosa Model: The brain metastasis volume of 8.28 cc carries a Volume Score VS=2. The histology small cell carcinoma carries a Radioresistance Score RS=1. The left petrous apex carries an Eloquence Score ES=2. Sosa Score will be SS=VS+RS+ES=2+1+2=5. The recommended Dose will be D=SS+10=5+10=15Gy.

Figure 5a(Transverse Cut)
73 y/o man, diagnosed 2 years ago with limited stage small cell lung carcinoma. Treated with chemotherapy and radiation therapy. Diplopia on left gaze starting a week ago.
Volume: 8.28cc. VS=2, RS=1, ES=2. SS= 5

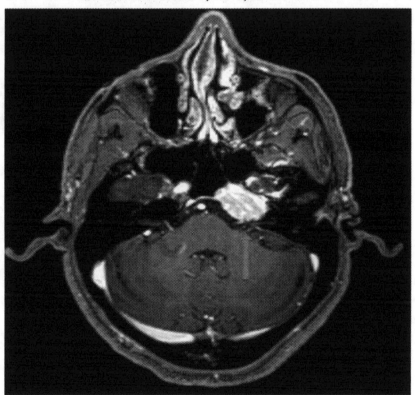

Metastasis of Small Cell Lung Carcinoma – Petrous Apex

Figure 5b(Coronal Cut)

Metastasis of Small Cell Lung Carcinoma

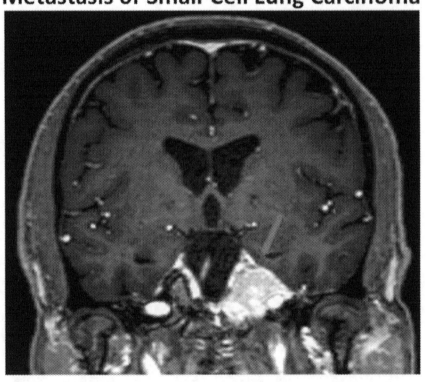

Figure 5c(Sagittal Cut)
Metastasis of Small Cell Lung Carcinoma

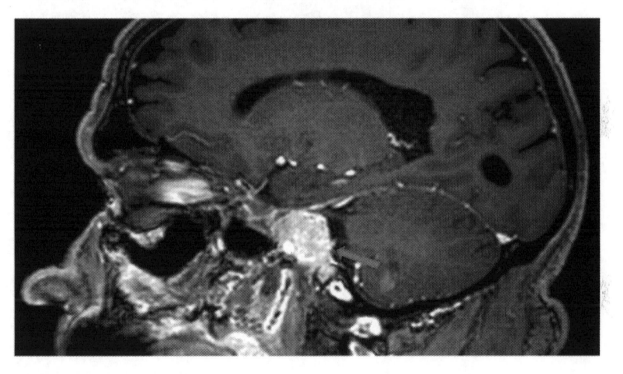

----CASE 6----

History: A 28 year old patient with history of renal transplantation 2 years ago, who is receiving systemic antirejection therapy, presents to her nephrologist clinic complaining of worsening headaches and right hemiparesis. An MRI (see Figures 6) shows a 3.14cc tumor consistent with low grade astrocytoma located in the left thalamus. She declines any consideration for craniotomy. The patient is sent to the neurosurgery clinic to be evaluated for GKRS.

Dose Determination Using the Sosa Model: A Tumor Volume of 3.14cc (between 0.01cc and 3.50cc) carries a VS=4. The Radioresistance Score of astrocytoma is RS=3. The Eloquence Score of the left thalamus is ES=1. Sosa Score=VS+RS+ES=4+3+1= 8. Recommended Dose=D=SS+10= 8+10=18 Gy.

Figure 6a(Transverse Cut)

28 y/o Lady, Headaches, Right Hemiparesis.
Volume:3.14cc. VS=4, RS=3, ES=1. SS= 8

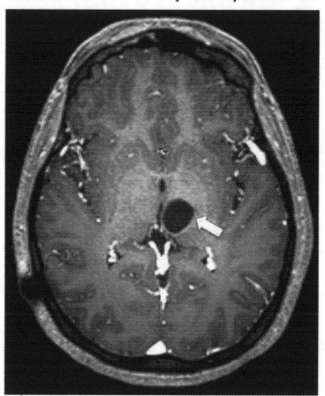

ASTROCYTOMA I – Left Thalamus

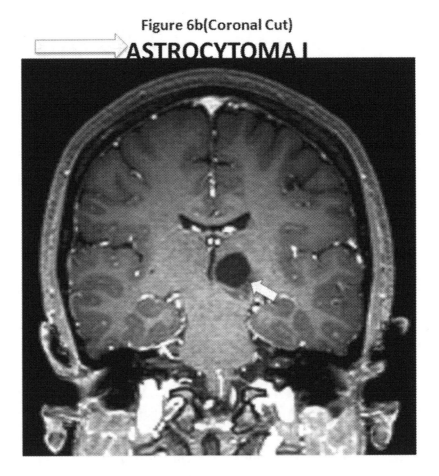

Figure 6b(Coronal Cut)
ASTROCYTOMA I

Figure 6c(Sagittal Cut)
ASTROCYTOMA I

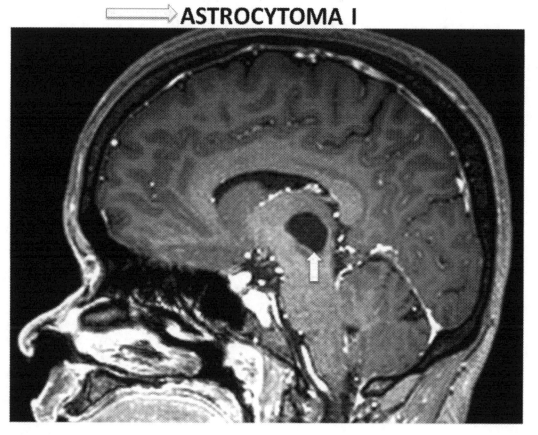

----CASE 7----

History: 88 year old lady diagnosed 5 months ago with Stage IIIB left breast poorly differentiated adenocarcinoma, ER and PR positive, Her2neu negative, was treated with mastectomy followed by radiation therapy. The patient did not receive any systemic therapy secondary to long history of DVT. She presented to her primary care practitioner a week ago with new onset of headaches. An MRI of the brain (see Figures 7) was pertinent for an 8.81cc mass consistent with metastasis located in the apex of the left superior frontal gyrus.

Dose Determination Using the Sosa Model: The brain metastasis volume of 8.81cc (between 7.01cc and 10.50cc) carries a VS=2. The histology of poorly differentiated adenocarcinoma carries a RS=2. The apex of the left superior frontal gyrus carries an ES=2. Sosa Score will be=2+2+2=6. Recommended Dose will be D=SS+10=16Gy. Please, note that both superior frontal gyruses have ES=2. There is a relatively low functionality associated to these areas; hence, ES=2 bilaterally.

Figure 7a(Sagittal Cut)

88 y/o Lady, Breast Ca.; Surgery+Radiation Completed 5 Months Ago.
VOLUME: 8.81cc.   VS=2, RS=2, ES=2. SS=6

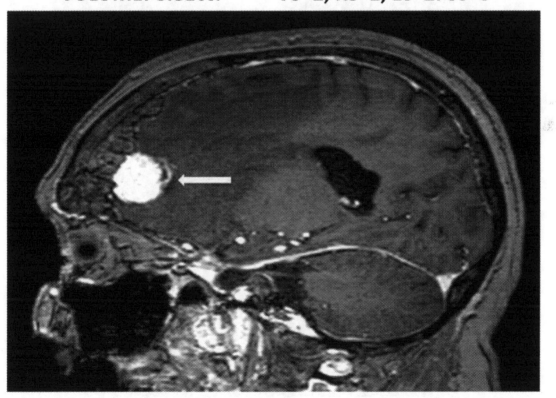

BREAST CANCER METASTASIS - Apex of the Left Superior Frontal Gyrus

Figure 7b(Transverse Cut)

BREAST CANCER METASTASIS

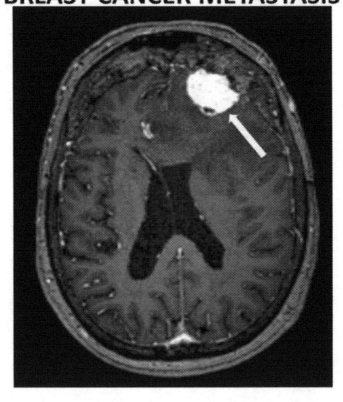

Figure 7c(Coronal Cut)

BREAST CANCER METASTASIS

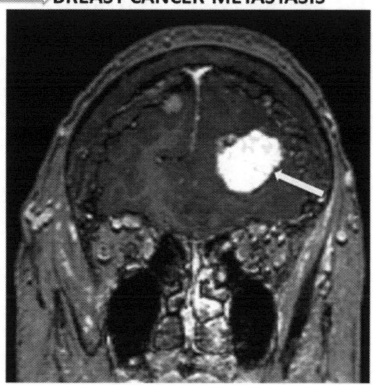

----CASE 8----

History: 66 year old frail gentleman presents to his primary care practitioner complaining of worsening headaches and fatigue. An MRI of the brain (see Figure 8) is pertinent for a 1.64 cc tumor suspicious for schwannoma located at the left pontocerebellar angle. The patient is referred to the neurosurgery clinic for consideration of Gamma Knife Radiation Surgery.

Dose Determination Using the Sosa Model: Volume Score (VS=4), Radioresistance Score (RS=3), Eloquence Score (ES=2). Sosa Score (SS)=VS+RS+ES=4+3+2=9. Recommended Dose: This is an "out of the box" case. Please review thoroughly CASE 1 where it was recommended for a Schwannoma located in the same "neurologic neighborhood" 15Gy for a tumor with Sosa Score=8. A simple extrapolation will lead to a recommendation of 16Gy Dose. This is a case in which the convenient formula (Dose= Sosa Score + 10) should NOT be applied. If you do not understand the reasoning behind this Recommended Dose, please review CASE 1 carefully.

Figure 8(Transverse Cut)

66 y/o Man, Headache and Fatigue.
Volume: 1.64cc.   VS=4, RS=3, ES=2. SS=9

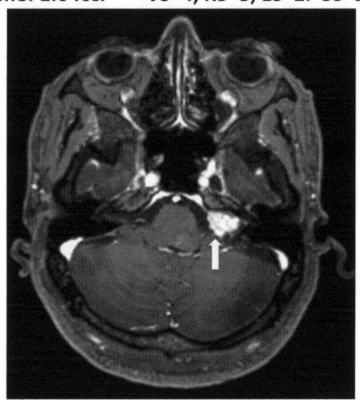

SCHWANNOMA – Pontocerebellar Angle

----CASE 9----

History: 47 year old lady diagnosed with Pituitary Null Cell Adenoma treated with transsphenoidal surgery 10 years ago, lost to follow for seven years, re-presents to neurosurgical clinic complaining of moderate fatigue; she wants "to know what is going on inside my head after so many years without seeing a doctor". Patient denies visual symptoms, headaches, dizziness, balance issues. Physical exam is within normal limits. A follow up MRI (see Figures 9) shows a recurrent mass, 4.69 cc in volume, occupying a portion of the surgical bed. Please, figure out GKRS dose.

Dose Determination Using the Sosa Model: Volume Score VS=3; Radioresistance Score RS=3; the pituitary locus Eloquence Score ES=1; Sosa Score=VS+RS+ES=3+3+1=7; the Recommended Dose will be D=SS+10=7+10=17Gy.

Figure 9a(Sagittal Cut)
47 y/o Lady, Pituitary Null Cell Adenoma, Transsphenoidal Surgery 10 years ago, Regrowth.
Volume: 4.69cc. VS= 3, RS=3, ES=1. SS= 7

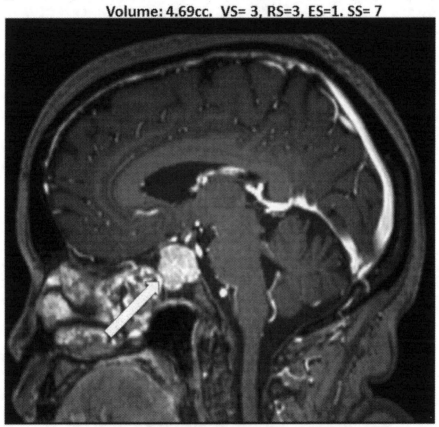

⟹ **Pituitary Null Cell Adenoma**

Figure 9b(Transverse Cut)

NULL CELL ADENOMA

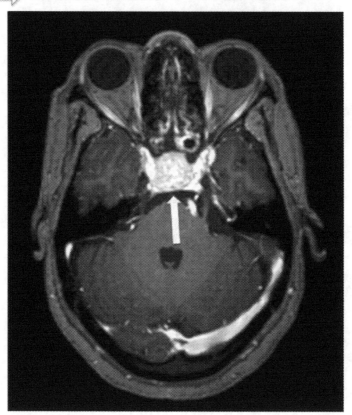

Figure 9c(Coronal Cut)

NULL CELL ADENOMA

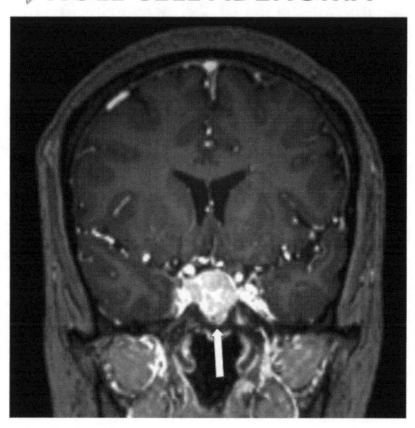

----CASE 10----

History: A 76 year old gentleman was diagnosed with Sphenoid Sinus Sarcoma 10 years ago. The patient was treated with transsphenoidal total macroscopic resection followed by external beam radiation therapy. He recovered nicely from treatment and was lost to follow up. He came back to the clinic feeling "very tired" and worrying about "having my head cancer back". Physical exam was within normal limits. A follow up MRI (see Figures 10), the first in 8 years secondary to patient's incompliance with follow up, was pertinent for a 21.71cc dominant mass consistent with recurrence in the petrous bone area. Patient consents to salvage Gamma Knife Radiation Surgery (GKRS) after being explained pros and cons of this procedure.

Dose Determination Using the Sosa Model: A tumor volume of 21.71cc carries a Volume Score VS=1. The sarcoma histology carries a Radioresistance Score RS=4. The tumor locus carries an Eloquence Score ES=2. Sosa Score is SS=VS+RS+ES=1+4+2=7. The Recommended Dose D=SS+10= 7+10=17Gy.

Figure 10a(Transverse Cut)
76 y/o Man. Operated 10 years ago of a Sphenoid Sinus Sarcoma. Regrowth.
Volume: 21.71cc . VS=1, RS=4, ES=2. SS= 7

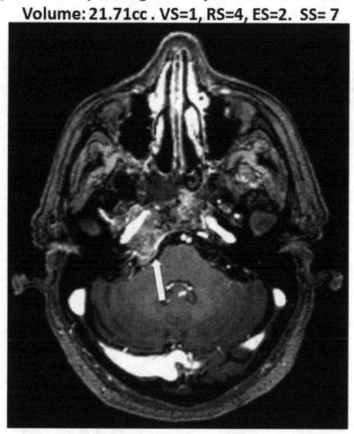

⟹ **SARCOMA – Petrous Bone**

Figure 10b(Coronal Cut)

SARCOMA

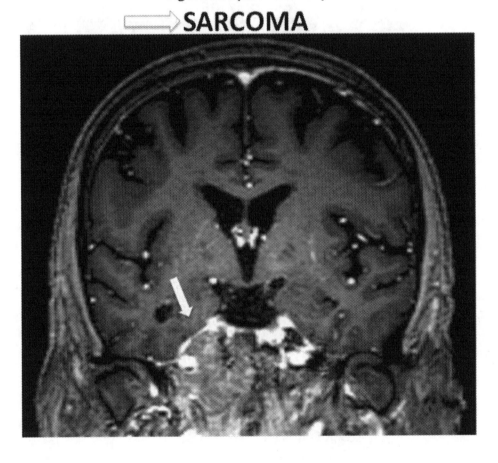

Figure 10c(Sagittal Cut)

SARCOMA

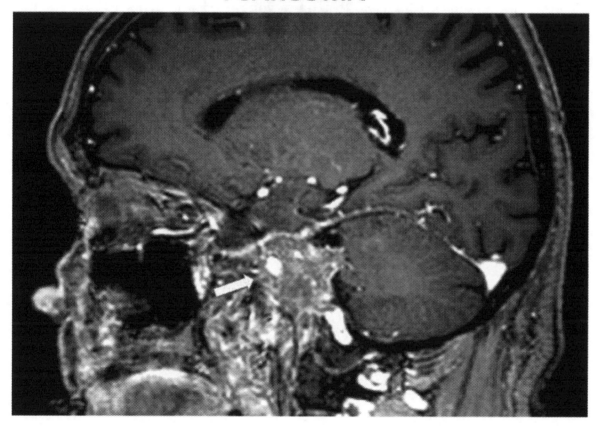

----CASE 11----

History: A 43 year old lady presents to her primary physician with worsening headaches not controlled by over the counter painkillers of 5 months evolution. An MRI of the brain (see Figures 11) is pertinent for an abnormal 0.77cc mass, located in the anterior third of the frontal interhemispheric cistern, very suggestive of meningioma. The patient declines any craniotomy option at the neurosurgery clinic and consents to GKRS.

Dose Determination Using the Sosa Model: Tumor volume 0.77cc carries a VS=4; meningioma carries a RS=3; tumor location carries an ES=3. Sosa Score=4+3+3=10. Recommended Dose= SS+10=10+10=20Gy.

Figure 11a(Transverse Cut)
Lady 43 y/o. New daily chronic headaches in the last several months.
Volume: 0.77cc   VS=4, RS=3, ES=3. SS=10

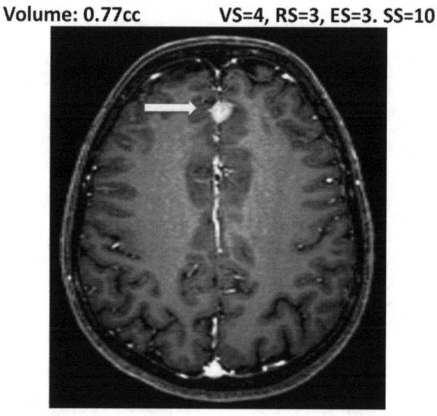

MENINGIOMA into the Anterior Third of the Frontal Interhemispheric Cistern

Figure 11b(Coronal Cut)

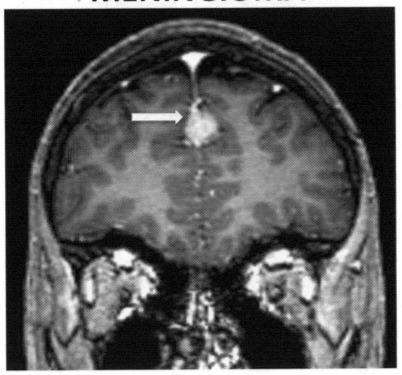

Figure 11c(Sagittal Cut)
⟹ MENINGIOMA

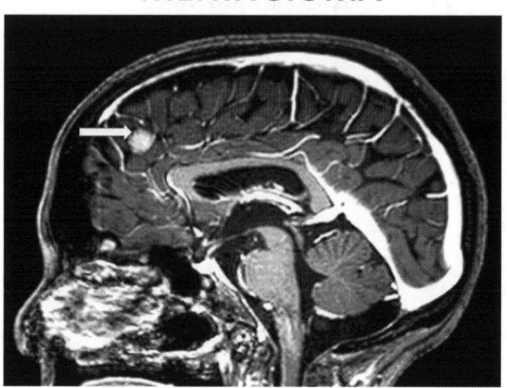

----CASE 12----

History: A 45 year old lady presented a year ago with a meningioma located in the right Rolandic area that was resected with minimal residual disease. Patient did well after craniotomy and was fine until a month ago, when she re-presented complaining of left gaze diplopia. An MRI of the brain (See Figures 12) was pertinent for a 0.88cc meningioma of the posterior pole of the left cavernous sinus. Patient consented to GKRS.

Dose Determination Using the Sosa Model: A tumor volume of 0.88cc carries a Volume Score VS=4. A meningioma carries a Radioresistance Score RS=3. The tumor location carries an Eloquence Score ES=2. Sosa Score SS=4+3+2=9. Recommended Dose D=SS+10=9+10=19 Gy.

**Figure 12a(Transverse Cut)
Lady 45 y/o. Left gaze diplopia recently.
Volume:0.88cc. VS=4, RS=3, ES=2. SS=9**

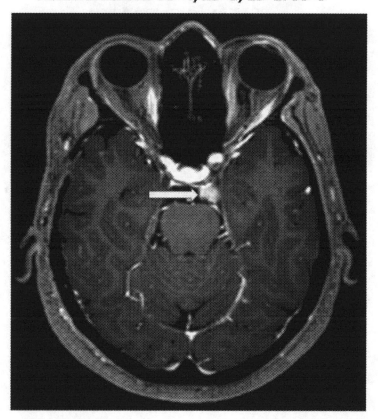

MENINGIOMA - Posterior Pole of the Left Cavernous Sinus

Figure 12b(Coronal Cut)

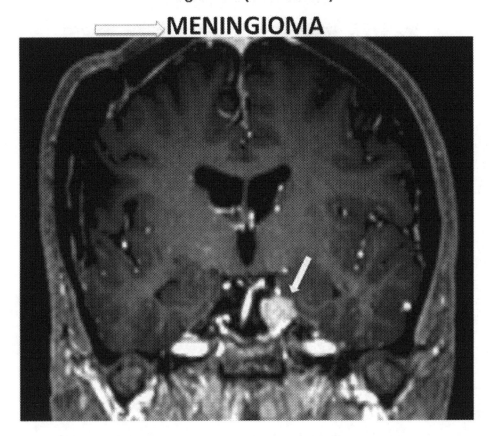

MENINGIOMA

Figure 12c(Sagittal Cut)
MENINGIOMA

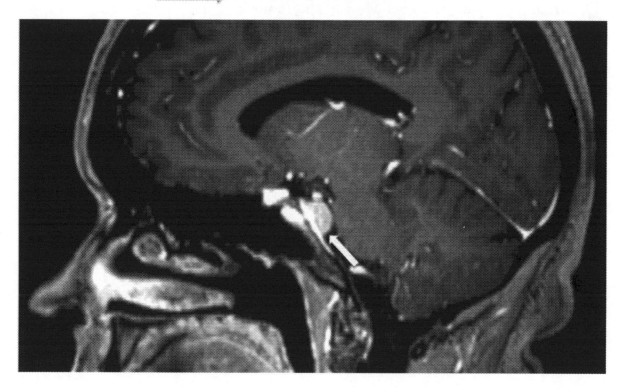

----CASE 13----

History: A 68 year old lady with no health problems besides hypertension and type 2 diabetes, well controlled on medications, presented a month ago to her primary practitioner complaining of focal motor seizures in the left leg and worsening headaches not controlled on over the counter pain killers. An MRI ordered at the neurosurgery clinic (see Figures 13) is pertinent for a 30.13cc meningioma located in the right paracentral lobe. The patient rejects any consideration for craniotomy and consents to GKRS.

Dose Determination Using the Sosa Model: The tumor volume of 30.13cc carries a Volume Score VS=1. Meningioma histology has a Radioresistance Score RS=3. The tumor location has an Eloquence Score ES=1. Sosa Score will be SS=VS+RS+ES=1+3+1=5. Recommended Dose will be D=SS+10= 5+10=15Gy. Note that several tumors evaluated in this chapter have volumes bigger than 14.00 cc and still can be treated following the Sosa Model (see discussion in the last few paragraphs of the chapter dedicated to Volume Score). Please, note that both paracentral lobes have ES=1.

Figure 13a(Transverse Cut)
68 y/o Lady. Focal motor seizures in the left leg and headaches for one month.
Volume: 30.13cc. VS=1, RS=3, ES=1. SS=5

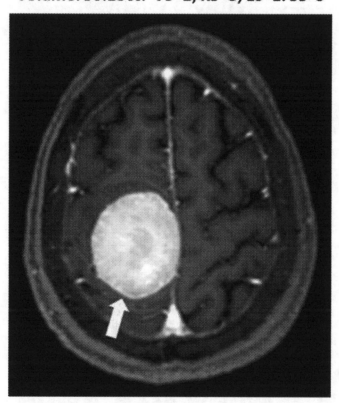

MENINGIOMA of the Right Paracentral Lobe

Figure 13b(Coronal Cut)

MENINGIOMA

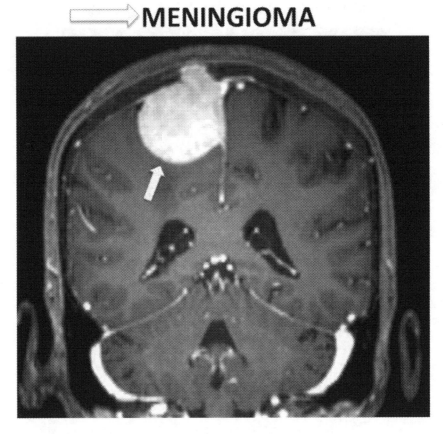

Figure 13c(Sagittal Cut)

MENINGIOMA

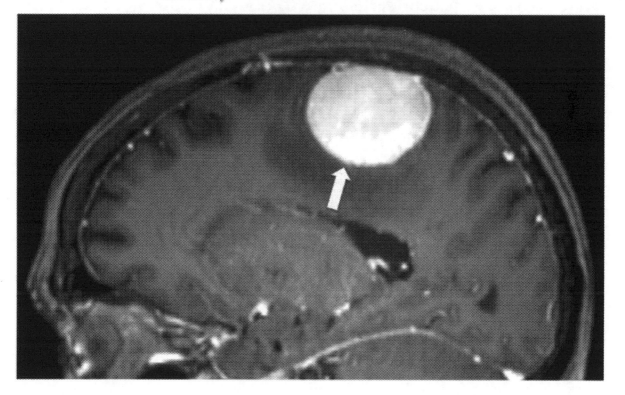

----CASE 14----

History: A 76 year old gentleman, with long standing smoking history and "healthy", presented a few weeks ago with seizures and headaches that prompted an MRI at an emergency room (see Figures 14) pertinent for a couple of small masses consistent with metastases; the biggest one, 0.68cc in volume, was located in the left globus pallidus and internal capsule. A CT scan of chest was pertinent for a neoplastic looking mass in the right lung upper lobe infiltrating the mediastinum; mediastinal lymph nodes in the ipsilateral paratracheal station are abnormal; a CT guided biopsy of the lung mass is consistent with poorly differentiated adenocarcinoma. The patient declines any consideration for surgery. The rest of radiological work up is negative. Please determine the most adequate Dose for the biggest and symptomatic brain metastasis.

Dose Determination Using the Sosa Model: A brain metastasis volume of 0.68cc carries a Volume Score VS=4. Histology of poorly differentiated adenocarcinoma carries a Radioresistance Score RS=2. The metastasis location carries an Eloquence Score ES=1. Sosa Score will be SS=VS+RS+ES=4+2+1=7. The recommended Dose will be D=SS+10=7+10=17Gy.

Figure 14a(Transverse Cut)

76 y/o Male. Heavy Smoker. Headaches, seizures and blurred vision. Lung cancer detected in Chest CT. Volume: 0.68cc.   VS=4, RS=2, ES=1. SS= 7

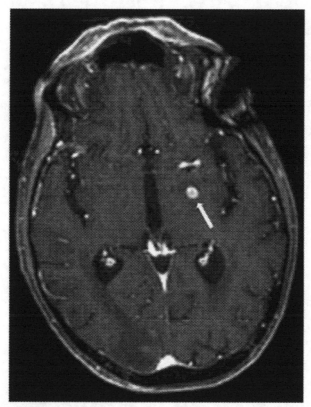

⟹ **LUNG CANCER METASTASIS** into the left Globus Pallidus and Internal Capsule

Figure 14b(Coronal Cut)

LUNG CANCER METASTASIS

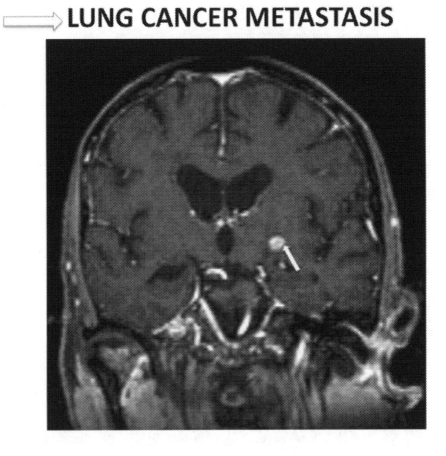

Figure 14c(Sagittal Cut)

LUNG CANCER METASTASIS

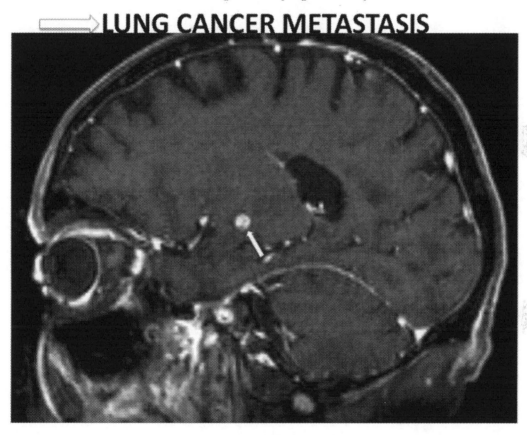

----CASE 15----

History: A 72 year old lady presents complaining of headache and left hemiparesis. An MRI of the brain (see Figures 15) reveals a gigantic right temporooccipital mass with a tentorium cerebelli component consistent with cancer that is treated with supratentorial resection; the pathologic diagnostic tests are consistent with hemangiopericytoma. A postoperatory follow up MRI reveals an enhancing 6.26cc mass consistent with a residual tumor implanted in the tentorium cerebelli. The patient discusses options and consents to GKRS.

Determination of Recommended Dose using the Sosa Model: The Volume Score corresponding to a tumor volume of 6.26cc is VS=3. Radioresistance Score for hemangiopericytoma is RS=4. The tumor locus carries an ES=4. Sosa Score is SS=VS+RS+ES=3+4+4=11. Recommended Dose D=SS+10=11+10=21Gy.

Figure 15a(Sagittal Cut)
72 y/o Lady. Right Temporooccipital mass is discovered.
A Tentorial implantation was evident in the post contrast MRI

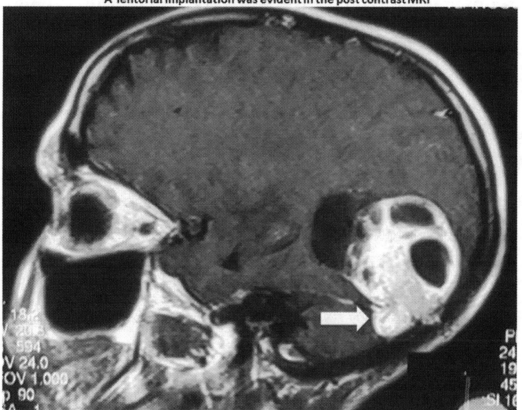

After supratentorial resection Immunohistochemistry showed Hemangiopericytoma

Figure 15 b(Sagittal Cut)
Remnant in Implantation is documented in MRI. Volume 6.26cc, VS=3. RS=4, ES=4. SS=11

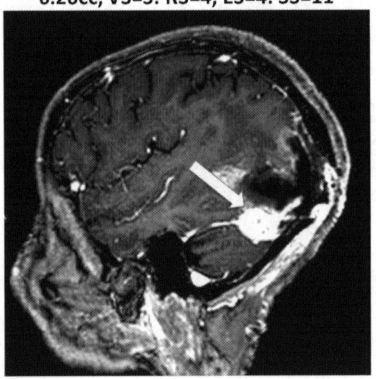

⟹ HEMANGIOPERICYTOMA – Tentorium Cerebelli

Figure 15 c(Transverse Cut)
HEMANGIOPERICYTOMA

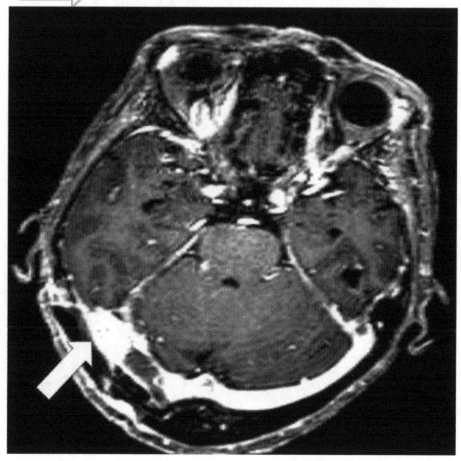

Figure 15d(Coronal Cut)   ⇒**HEMANGIOPERICYTOMA**

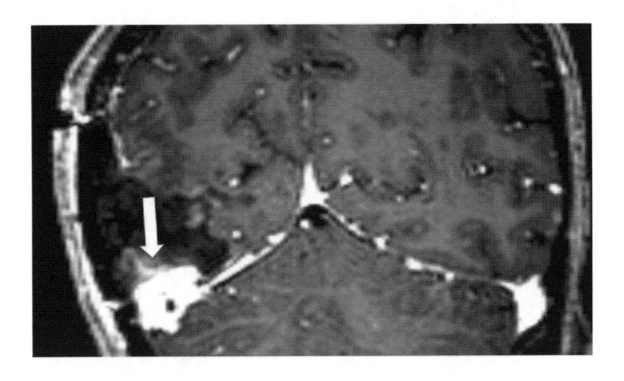

----CASE 16----

History: A 76 year old gentleman with 60 years smoking history of one pack a day presents to his primary care practitioner with headaches, blurred vision and one incident of seizures. An MRI of the brain (see Figures 16) is pertinent for an 8.06cc suspicious mass localized at the right superior parietal gyrus. A CT scan of the chest demonstrates a mass in the right lung upper lobe and multiple enlarged mediastinal lymph nodes. CT guided biopsy of the lung mass is reported by pathology as consistent with poorly differentiated squamous cell carcinoma of the right lung. The patient declines any consideration for craniotomy at the neurosurgery clinic and consents to GKRS.

Determination of Dose Using the Sosa Model: A brain metastasis volume of 8.06cc carries a Volume Score VS=2. The histology of squamous cell carcinoma carries a Radioresistance Score RS=2. The metastasis location carries an Eloquence Score ES=1. The Sosa Score for this metastasis is SS=VS+RS+ES=2+2+1=5. The Dose will be D=SS+10=5+10=15Gy. Note that the ES=1 even though the lesion is located in the non-dominant brain hemisphere. This is so because the superior parietal gyrus, bilaterally, regulates the important function of tactile perception and recognition of the shape of objects (stereognosis), which is prone to be affected as a result of GKRS.

Figure 16a(Transverse Cut)
76 y/o Male. Heavy Smoker. Headache, seizures and blurred vision. Lung cancer
detected in Chest CT. Volume: 8.06cc. VS=2, RS=2, ES=1. SS= 5

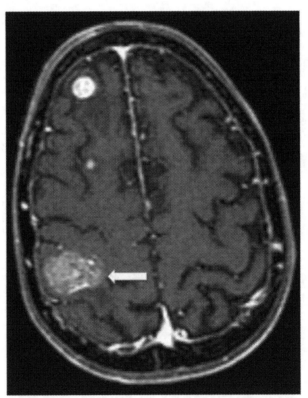

⇨ LUNG CANCER METASTASIS - Right Superior Parietal Gyrus

Figure 16b(Coronal Cut)

LUNG CANCER METASTASIS

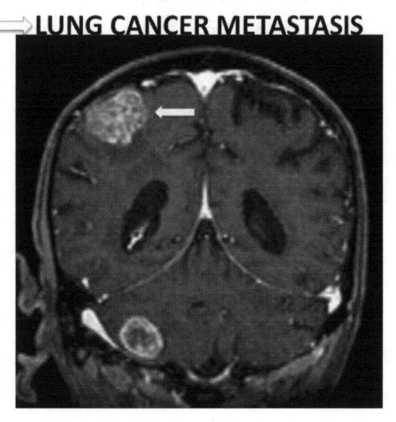

Figure 16c(Sagittal Cut)

LUNG CANCER METASTASIS

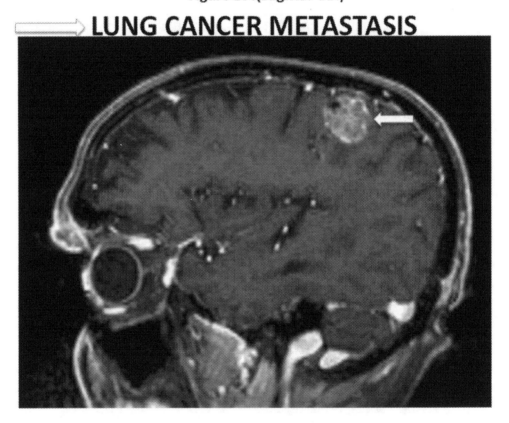

----CASE 17----

History: A 47 year old lady who had GKRS for an acoustic neuroma 6 months ago presented for a follow up at her radiosurgery clinic. An MRI (see Figures 17) showed an abnormality, located between the two paracentral lobes, consistent with a 0.69cc meningioma. Observation was recommended in view of the lack of symptoms. The patient, one week after this finding, represented to the clinic complaining of excruciating headache not relieved with full doses of over the counter painkillers. She was started on opioids that caused nausea, dizziness and constipation. The patient discussed options, declined any consideration for craniotomy and consented to GKRS for her meningioma.

Determination of Dose Using the Sosa Model: The tumor volume of 0.69cc carries a Volume Score VS=4. The histology of meningioma carries a Radioresistance Score RS=3. The tumor location carries an Eloquence Score ES=1. Sosa Score will be SS=VS+RS+ES=4+3+1=8. The Recommended Dose will be D=SS+10=8+10=18Gy.

Figure 17a(Sagittal Cut)
47 y/o Lady. Follow up MRI 6 months after GKRS for Acoustic Neuroma. Incidental finding.
Volume: 0.69cc. VS=4, RS=3,ES=1. SS=8

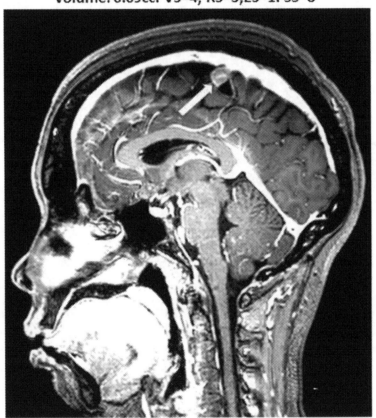

MENINGIOMA between the two Paracentral Lobes

Figure 17b(Transverse Cut)
MENINGIOMA

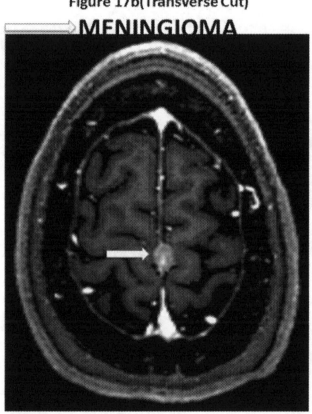

Figure 17 c(Coronal Cut)

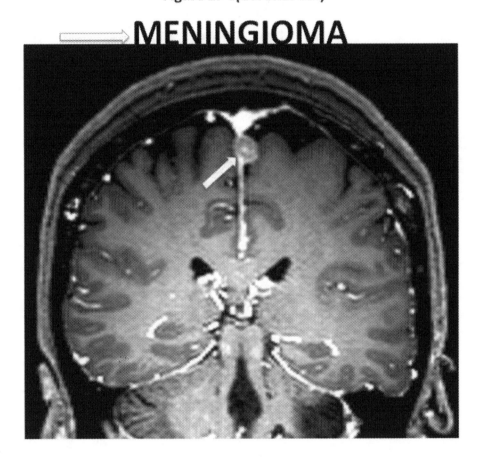

MENINGIOMA

CHAPTER SEVEN

REFLECTIONS AND CONCLUSIONS

After presenting in detail a new paradigm for the determination of doses used in Gamma Knife Radiation Surgery, the author feels it is necessary to share with the reader some aspects of the process that led to its conception and to reflect on some of its features.

The first thing that should be clear is that this intellectual effort is not the product of improvisation. The author conceived the Sosa Model in 2001 and made, while working in GKRS during the last 10 years, several attempts to perform retrospective studies that could have tested his model, starting with the validation of the Volume Score (VS). Those research proposals were greeted with initial sympathy in several institutions, but when they reached the level of legal clearance, very understandably, they flunked.

It would be just reasonable that a legal department consulted regarding a research project anticipated to evaluate the accuracy of the doses administered in a Gamma Knife center would raise a red flag. The retrospective validation of the Volume Score contained in the Sosa Model (SM) could potentially have opened a box full of liability worms that could have impacted negatively the finances of a Gamma Knife center just at the peak of the biggest crisis in the world economy in the last 80 years.

What should a responsible physician do when he sees the product of his hypothesis building process vetoed for very understandable reasons? Should he shut his intellect and engage in activities more attractive for a person approaching retirement age like golf or touring? Or should he simply live on a day to day basis until he witnesses a model similar to his being proposed by another curious medical specialist impressed by the lack of rigor that has characterized the determination of doses in GKRS since the genius of Dr. Leksell gave birth to the wonder of scientific creativity embodied in a Gamma Knife unit?

The creator of the Sosa Model rejected the two options mentioned in the precedent paragraph, and decided to share his invention with every single human being interested in the miracle of radiosurgery through the magic of the electronic book industry that has made possible to many thousands of authors with limited financial resources, like himself, to submit to the consideration of the global public their ideas, projects and dreams.

The importance of the suitability and reproducibility of the doses applied to intracranial tumors in GKRS should not be underestimated. If a given tumor receives a dose lower than the one capable to control it, the unsuited low dose will increase the chances of tumor progression. On the other hand, if a tumor located in a very delicate area receives a dose higher than the one tolerated by its locus the chances of GKRS toxicities increase considerably.

Who do you think would estimate doses more adequately and reproducibly, a radiosurgery specialist that takes into consideration the tumor histology and the eloquence of the tumor location, or one that basically ignores those variables? One who takes into consideration the tumor volume or one that substitutes a shaky maximum diameter for the tumor volume? The answer is left to the reader's common sense.

A flawless GKRS unit will NOT do the best job possible if the doses used are not calculated optimally. At this point, we have to remind ourselves that many specialists treating patients with GKRS are not veterans in the art of radiosurgery.

When experience is not present in clinical practice, standardization is paramount for attaining quality. How can we pretend to have top quality GKRS without standardizing the way to figure out GKRS doses?

The day that we have a model, either the Sosa Model or another one which proves to be superior, that can guide the radiosurgical practitioners in the process of choosing the optimal dose for intracranial tumors taking into consideration relevant variables like Volume, Radioresistance and Eloquence, we will be comfortable with the clinical quality control in GKRS. As long as we do NOT have such a methodology up and running in the hundreds of GKRS units working all over the world, there will be an unfinished homework for the radiosurgical community.

Gamma Knife Radiation Surgery (GKRS) was conceived, delivered and nurtured in Sweden and settled in several continents before moving to the USA when it was almost 40 years old. This means that the theoretical base of GKRS was not built in the USA.

As we have said before, while the GKRS units have improved technically tremendously since its invention, to the point of naming the most sophisticated GK model "Perfexion", the theoretical base to determine the doses to be administered in GKRS has not experienced substantial changes since its birth.

The evident imbalance in progress between theory and practice in GKRS does not do any good to this discipline. As of 2015, GKRS is an empiric specialty based on the accumulation of data coming from a laborious heuristic clinical activity; its scientific base is still somewhat blurred. The best time to initiate a process that can change this situation is now, when solid retrospective data is showing that fractionated GKRS is not only feasible, but pretty effective in the management of tumors in the close vicinity of the optic apparatus and when we are getting closer to admitting that GKRS is not out of the realm of radiobiology.

The research that will lead to a new paradigm for determination of doses in GKRS will most probably take place outside the USA. As we have said before, the practice of medicine in the USA has legal risks for the use of data that could potentially show that old methods in dose determination in GKRS could have caused morbidity in some patients. A study showing superiority of a new model, like the Sosa Model, compared to the status quo, could put any Gamma Knife center in the USA in a really problematic financial situation.

What would be the research proposal that the Sosa Model inventor would make to several Gamma Knife centers in the future? This proposal is rather simple; its first stage will be to perform a retrospective study to validate or discard the maximum diameter as surrogate for the tumor volume in a couple of thousands of tumors treated with GKRS. If this retrospective analysis shows the maximum diameter to be an inadequate surrogate for the tumor volume in GKRS, it would be followed by a prospective, randomized, stratified (Phase III) trial comparing the results of GKRS in 2 arms: one using the status quo methodology, and another one using the Sosa Model for Determination of Doses in GKRS.

Is it important, or even relevant, to determine accurately the radiosurgical doses delivered to patients that in most cases are destined to die in a matter of months or, in the best scenario, in a few years? Whoever responds negatively the precedent question does not understand the ethical base of medicine. We, physicians, are obligated to make every single effort to improve the care that we deliver to our patients, and treating radiosurgery patients with doses produced by a methodology built on a shaky heuristic iteration process could have been satisfactory a few decades ago, but not in 2015, when the rudimentary first generation GK units are museum pieces. Who could feel safe flying in a Boeing 777 under the command of a pilot who insists in using the Polar star instead of computerized navigation systems for orientation in the sky during a perilous transatlantic trip?

The author is fully aware of the multiple limitations of the Sosa Model. To depict an intracranial tumor as a mix of Volume, Radioresistance and Eloquence is, in the best scenario, a gross approximation to a much more complex reality. That being said, this model, the Sosa Model, is much closer to reality than substituting a maximum tumor diameter for a tumor volume and ignoring tumor histology and location inside the cranium, which is what the status quo does, as far as dose determination in radiosurgery, in most cases.

Regarding the Volume Score (VS), the Sosa Model divides in four quartiles the possible volume values and assigns to them VS values of positive integers from 1 to 4. This is a gross approximation to a much more complex reality where not all volume values have the same probability to occur. A more accurate way to assign VS values would be to perform a retrospective study with thousands of intracranial tumors amenable to radiosurgery and, using complex statistical tools that the author, frankly speaking, does not have the command of, to group intracranial tumors in more representative quartiles.

The quartiles suggested by the Sosa Model (see Volume Score chapter) are crutches that this new model needs to stand up and walk. The day a more representative tumor distribution is available, as a result of the above suggested study, the Sosa model would be able to RUN, not simply to walk. In the author's opinion, a medium size GKRS center with a couple of thousands of tumors on file could room the needed retrospective study.

An argument can be made for the TUMOR EXTERNAL AREA, rather than the TUMOR VOLUME, to be a surrogate for the number of normal intracranial cells affected by radiosurgery. This argument is particularly strong in the case of EXPANDING tumors, like benign meningiomas, that push normal surrounding structures without infiltrating them. The reality today is that most GKRS units are able to measure tumor VOLUME and not TUMOR EXTERNAL AREA. In addition to this, many tumors expand and infiltrate simultaneously while they grow. In future, when we could have the capacity of measuring the TUMOR EXTERNAL AREA, this could be a fascinating topic to research.

Regarding Radioresistance Score (RS), histology is a discipline in constant change. It should be expected that the assigned RS for multiple tumors could vary. These variations would alter Sosa Score for those tumors, but will leave the Sosa Model intact; because every tumor will still be able to be assigned a Radioresistance Score

(RS) integer from 1 to 4. If a GKRS specialist disagrees at the present time with a particular value contained in the RS Table displayed in the Radioresistance Score chapter, he can still use the Sosa Model in his clinic, changing the RS as he deems appropriate, to determine radiosurgical doses.

Last, but not least, the Eloquence Scores (ES) of multiple intracranial loci are liable to vary in future if we accept the premise that neurosciences are rapidly evolving disciplines. The author feels very comfortable with the Eloquence Score scale used in this book, considering the outstanding qualifications of its creator Santiago Valenzuela Sosa MD. On the other hand, in science, as in life, change is, as Heraclitus taught us, a constant. But even assuming future changes in the assignment of Eloquence Scores to multiple intracranial loci, those locations will be able to be assigned a positive integer ES from 1 to 4.

Bottom line, accepting the fact that the parameters VS, RS and ES are far from perfection and liable to experience changes in the positive integers (1 to 4) that describe them for different tumors, we will still be able to have a Sosa Score with a minimum value of 3 and a maximum value of 12 that will be useful in alleviating the unnecessary anxiety that today many radiosurgery specialists experience at the time of assigning doses in their clinics.

If we get to the point that, when presented with a new radiosurgery case, the specialist in charge is able to figure out quickly the tumor VOLUME, HISTOLOGY AND LOCUS and to assign appropriate VS, RS and ES; and then he adds those parameters to obtain a Sosa Score (SS) that will easily lead to a recommended Dose, we will feel that we have accomplished a small but crucial step in the necessary process of clinical optimization of radiosurgery.

It is worthwhile to remind the reader that the Sosa Model is NOT proposing to change the range of doses used in GKRS and is NOT suggesting to use any new device not available at the present time in a standard GKRS suite. What the Sosa Model proposes is to CUSTOMIZE the radiosurgical doses using meaningful, universally reproducible and easily describable variables like tumor VOLUME,

HISTOLOGY AND INTRACRANIAL LOCUS. In other words, the Sosa Model is trying to OPTIMIZE and STANDARDIZE the way doses are calculated in GKRS; so complications caused by excessively high doses and recurrences facilitated by unnecessarily low doses are minimized.

It is expected, thank God, that systemic therapy will increase its effectiveness in the next few decades and eventually will convert different varieties of cancer, that are today lethal, to chronic conditions comparable, as far as prognosis, with diabetes and rheumatoid arthritis. At that time, cancer patients treated with radiosurgery could feel the impact of the use of an outdated methodology in figuring out their GKRS doses. Any effort that we make today in improving the adequacy and reproducibility of doses in radiosurgery will be reflected tomorrow in increased benefits and reduced toxicities in brains and other intracranial structures touched by Gamma rays.

Hopefully, the publication of the Sosa Model will awake the interest of many brilliant scientists involved in radiosurgery who will revise, correct and improve this humble effort of pushing the borders of the theoretical base of dose determination in GKRS.

The author thanks very much those who have read this book and hopes that the ideas contained in it excite the imagination of neurosurgeons, radiation oncologists, medical physicists, residents, medical students and others involved in radiosurgery.

Without the imagination of a genius like Dr. Leksell, millions of patients would have suffered much more the rigors of intracranial tumors. Let the imagination of many Dr. Leksell followers in the global village promote the real "perfection" of his dreams. If this model, which contains imperfections that will be corrected by the next generation of radiosurgeons all over the world, inspires its readers to challenge ideas pertaining to the initial stages of radiosurgery that are accepted today as sacred truths, following the Law of Inertia that is so prevailing in medical training in our era, the author would feel that the mental energy and the time invested in building the Sosa Model have been entirely justified.

REFERENCES

Andisheh B et al; Improving the therapeutic ratio in stereotactic radiosurgery: optimizing treatment protocols based on kinetics of repair of sublethal radiation damage; Technol Cancer Research Treat 2013 Aug 12(4):349-61.

Boari N et al; Gamma knife radiosurgery for vestibular schwannoma; J Neurosurgery 2014 Dec, 121 Suppl:123-42.

Deacon et al; Cited in Introduction to radiobiology by Dutreix et Al; CRC Press 1990 p.199.

Flickinger J et al; A multi-institutional experience with stereotactic radiosurgery for solitary brain metastasis; Int Radiat Oncol Biol Phys; 1994 Mar 1;28(4):797-802.

Jee TK et al; Fractionated gamma knife radiosurgery for benign perioptic tumors: outcome of 38 patients in a single institution; Brain Tumor Res Treat; 2014 Oct;2(2):56-61.

Nguyen, JH et al; Multisession gamma knife radiosurgery; World Neurosurg. 2014 Dec. 82(6): 1256-63.

Rubin P et al; Clinical radiation pathology; Philadelphia, W.B. Sanders, 1968.

Woo HJ et al; Factors related to the local treatment failure of gamma knife radiosurgery for metastatic brain tumors; Acta Neuruchir (Wein) 2010 Nov;152(11): 1909-14.

Printed in the United States
By Bookmasters